Spirituality and Mental Health
Breakthrough

Editors' Note

Originally, this book was to be edited by David Brandon and Phil Barker. Sadly, David died in 2001, as work was beginning on the book. Fortunately, he had completed one of his chapters for the book, 'Chocolate Cakes', which is published here.

It was our privilege to have taken over the editing of the book, and we hope that we have remained true to the spirit of the text that David first envisaged.

Spirituality and Mental Health
Breakthrough

Breakthrough

Edited by

PHIL BARKER PhD, RN, FRCN
Trinity College, Dublin

and

POPPY BUCHANAN-BARKER
Director, Clan Unity International, Fife

W

WHURR PUBLISHERS
LONDON AND PHILADELPHIA

© 2004 Whurr Publishers Ltd
First published 2004
by Whurr Publishers Ltd
19b Compton Terrace
London N1 2UN, England and
325 Chestnut Street, Philadelphia PA 19106, USA

British Library Cataloguing in Publication Data

A catalogue record for this book
is available from the British Library.

ISBN 1 86156 392 2

Contents

Chapter 13   **191**

Chapter 14   **200**

PART FIVE: **In the Long Shadow – In the Light**   **209**

Chapter 15   **211**

Dedication

This book is dedicated to the memories of our friends and family members who died during the production of this book, but especially Professor Steve Baldwin, Phyllis Barker, Frank Girvan, Professor Annie T Altschul and Professor David Brandon.

They all taught us much about the comfort of friendship and the sadness of loss. Representing both *something* and *nothing*, they reminded us of the enigma of the Self.

Be ye lamps unto yourselves.
Be your own reliance.
Hold to the truth within yourselves.
As to the only lamp.
Buddha

Lady Giladriel's Skin
by Gary Platz

We sat and spoke of Lunacy
This seventeen-year-old girl and I
The real thing
Not just a brown eye from a car
Lunch-time Lambton Quay

She said
I was standing naked on the window ledge
When he saw me
Screaming at the moon
For turning my arms silver
How could I jump
With Lady Giladriel's skin

I said
I was the Prince of Peace
Right here in the valley
Till I chucked it in
The pressure
Just hell on relationships

She said
He was quite nice at first
The one who saved me
But he turned out to be an alien
I have discovered that there has been some sort of invasion
My life has been all laser beams and black holes ever since

I said
Too many people
Things I had to do so right
And God the way he does
Said don't worry perhaps some other time

She said
One stood over me
Right there on the ward
While I was on my bed
Te Whare Ahuru*
I would rather die than go back to you

I said
I don't think I could be overtaken
By anything I didn't want to do
For I once gave up everything
Because I had too much to lose

She said
It's not so bad now I can tell the difference
There is something in the way they smile
I can walk down the street and say
They haven't got you
Not yet anyway

I said
I know there is a God of free will
For without choices who could I possibly be
Imagine me being the Prince of Peace
Imagine the Prince of Peace
Choosing to become me

She said
Te Whare Ahuru
I would rather live than go back to you
I think I will search through all I have
Maybe make something new
Something I will feel comfortable in
Something to compliment
My Lady Giladriel skin

---

* Te Whare Ahuru (*Tea far-e a-hu-ru*) is the local psychiatric ward. It means something like
  The house of calm healing.

Contributors

Phil Barker was the UK's first Professor of Psychiatric Nursing Practice, at the University of Newcastle, and is presently Visiting Professor at Trinity College, Dublin. He is a director of Clan Unity, the International Mental Health Recovery Agency, and is a psychotherapist. www.tidal-model.co.uk

Ian Beech teaches psychiatric nursing at the University of Glamorgan in South Wales and also works clinically with people in depression. He hopes that he may, in some small way, help people on their journey of recovery.

David Brandon was Professor of Community Care at Anglia Polytechnic University in Cambridge. He was the renowned author of over 200 books and academic papers, and was a popular speaker in public and on the radio. He was also a Buddhist monk.

Toby Brandon has a PhD from the London School of Economics, and is a senior lecturer in disability studies at the University of Northumbria and a senior research associate at the Centre for Applied Social Studies at the University of Durham.

Poppy Buchanan-Barker is managing director of Clan Unity, the International Mental Health Recovery Agency. She was a social worker for 26 years and has a background in counselling and advocacy. www.clan-unity.co.uk

Liam Clarke is a well-known Irish author and academic, and is presently senior lecturer in mental health nursing at the University of Brighton, England.

Sally Clay calls herself a 'recovering lunatic'. She works as a freelance writer and editor, sending attachments from her computer in central Florida, USA, to all points of the globe. Her writings are posted at http://home.earthlink.net/~sallyclay

Cathy Conroy is a former mental health advocate from Goulburn, New South Wales. She returned to classroom teaching last year after a break of 24 years. She also does voluntary welfare work with the St Vincent de Paul Society.

Larry Culliford has been a consultant psychiatrist in the NHS since 1988. He trained in medicine at Cambridge University and Guy's Hospital, and in psychiatry in New Zealand, South Australia and at St George's Hospital Medical School, London. He is involved with the 'Spirituality and Psychiatry' Special Interest Group of the Royal College of Psychiatrists.

Anne Drysdale is a daughter, sister, wife, mother, carer, singer, dabbler in art, Christian and graduate of the university of life.

Sue Holt worked for social services in England and then spent much of the past five years as a patient in psychiatric hospital. Presently she helps to produce a users' newsletter and also is a member of a user/carer training team.

Eibhlin Inglesby lives with her family in the north-east of England, and has worked as a nurse, and a teacher of nursing and theology.

Kenneth Leech is an Anglican priest, author and old friend and colleague of David Brandon. Since 1958 he has spent most of his time working in the East End of London.

Gary Platz is a person living with the experience of mental illness. Married with three children, Gary is a mental health consultant and director of Case Consulting Ltd and consumer advisor to Wellink Trust in New Zealand.

Nikki Slade is an actress and musician, presently living in London, where she provides workshops for a wide range of people through her agency, Free the Inner Voice.

Peter Wilkin is a psychiatric nurse, with special interests in clinical supervision and psychotherapy, presently living and working in Lancashire, England.

Foreword

TOBY BRANDON ON HIS FATHER DAVID

My father first became aware of mental illness at an early age. His own father's problems and the lack of care from the local hospital made him painfully acknowledge a need for greater insight. His father's violence towards him, and his own difficulties, forced him further down that path, first as a Quaker then later as a Zen Buddhist. He sometimes spoke to me about his identification with wounded healing and shamanism. Qualifying at the London School of Economics as a psychiatric social worker, he worked with people in many, often unconventional, ways. Mostly he saw the ability to stay in the present moment as a major component of mental wellness. 'Now' being the only time when we can actually do anything. To what extent can we bring our perception and energies into what is happening all around us? How much energy seeps away into anxiety, apprehension and guilt? We can sometimes hardly see or hear others in the 'noise' created by this muddle. This is both relevant to our own personal experience and vital to any kind of help we may give to others. Dad saw through many of the illusions of the self, which we try to create from the many different moments we experience. There is a Buddhist parable that illustrates how he tried to live his life:

A man travelling across a field encountered a tiger after him. Coming to a precipice, he caught hold of a root of a wild vine and swung himself down over the edge. The tiger sniffed at him from above. Trembling, the man looked down to where, far below, another tiger was waiting to eat him. Only the vine sustained him.

Two mice, one white and one black, little by little started to gnaw away the vine. The man saw a luscious strawberry near him. Grasping the vine with one hand, he picked the strawberry with the other. How sweet it tasted!

Reps (1971)

By trying to live in the moment and really be in that moment with others gave Dad the capability of a smart bomb homing in on peoples' troubles, no matter how deep their bunkers. To be the target of this could be both uncomfortable and funny. Dad found humour a great tool with which to teach and to learn, seeing life as so serious it should not be taken too seriously. The Dalai Lama always seems to be smiling. The passion with which Dad approached mental health was sometimes mistaken as a sign of a rampant ego. He observed that survivors of psychiatric services are often seen as loud, emotional beings in contrast to the calm, dispassionate mental health professionals. By acting out he bridged this gap.

My memories of his Buddhism are mixed. It made it hard for me to rebel as a teenager – it's troublesome having a robe-wearing, shaven-headed Dad, who is more 'out there' than you would like to be. I toyed with the idea of becoming a Christian but never quite went through with it. The Zendo (Zen Buddhist temple), which was a converted garage attached to our large Victorian house, attracted a growing number of people interested in Buddhism. They would wander around our garden in walking meditation and chant for hours. This chapter in our lives closed when my parents moved to a tiny flat in Cambridge. Dad never wanted to be a guru anyway.

My father was strongly against spiritual materialism, that pick-'n'-mix culture where people construct their spiritual being by taking a bit of Taoism, a dash of Buddhism and a little bit of whatever else they fancied. He saw this 'faddy' approach as lazy and not mindful, mindfulness not being about the pursuit of any intellectualism but just retaining the self-discipline to question. I believe this Zen self-discipline in many ways kept him alive through his troubled periods.

My mother nursed my father at home for the last five months of his life and she tells me that they were forced to live only in the moment because they had nothing else. They both were clinging to that vine together. He died in November 2001. His funeral was Buddhist but not a full-on affair with chanting and incense waving. That's not the kind of Buddhist he was in life. Spirituality to him was not about fuss but was a practical thing; it was about a disciplined commitment to helping yourself to help others. The cornerstone of this was the ability to ask the 'why' questions. For instance, in mental health: Why do we treat people like this? Does it really have to be this way?

Toby Brandon, Durham, 2003

Reference

Reps P (1971) Zen Flesh, Zen Bones. New York: Penguin.

Preface

POPPY BUCHANAN-BARKER AND PHIL BARKER

We're not our skin of grime, we're not our dread bleak dusty imageless locomotive, we're all golden sunflowers inside, blessed by our own seed & hairy naked accomplishment-bodies growing into mad black formal sunflowers in the sunset, spied on by our eyes under the shadow of the mad locomotive riverbank sunset Frisco hilly tincan evening sitdown vision.

From *Sunflower Sutra*, by Allen Ginsberg

Given our long association with the fields of 'mental health' and 'spirituality', we believe that this book will enlighten, disturb and frustrate, although perhaps not in that order. It may well be necessary for the reader to be sufficiently frustrated to become disturbed so that, ultimately, a whiff of the heady aroma of enlightenment might be possible.

If our experience is anything to go by, the journey towards understanding, if not actual enlightenment, often seems like 99% perspiration, although inspiration is also necessary. Indeed, the more difficult the journey becomes, the more we puff and blow, metaphorically – hence the more we need to *inspire*. But the sheer hard work of the journey is what we *feel*. Inspiration we take for granted. Like many other important aspects of being human, the spiritual life is built on a paradox. We struggle to *do* something – achieve understanding or enlightenment – that we should just allow to *come* to us. However, if we do not make the effort – if we do not commit ourselves; if we do not let ourselves *go* – the gift we seek will not *come*.

This paradoxical world of the Spirit seems like the right place to open this book. *Spirituality* is pretty much like breathing – betraying its Latin origins. *Spiritus* means, literally, the *breath* (of life). Throughout the course of our lives, the breath washes in, through and out of our bodies, like twenty thousand daily waves. With each inhalation we sound an echo of our first breath, which whispered our entry into the world. With each exhalation, we rehearse the final breath, when we shall finally release our fragile grip on life and, at least, the physical living of it. The breath of life enters us, almost unbidden, and certainly takes its leave of us without per-mission. However hard we try to control our breathing – through the rigours of yoga or one of the many forms of meditation – invariably we learn that we might be better off simply *watching*. If we have learned any-thing of any note about our own spiritual lives, this is it.

Listen, watch and learn. Everything else is mere wallpaper.

Spirituality has always been with us, if not in the practice of everyday life, then at least within the various religious traditions and their philo-sophical backgrounds. However, spirituality as a discrete *idea*, if not a movement, caught fire in the final decade of the 20th century. To a great extent this reflected the widespread anticipation of spiritual fireworks at the imaginary Millennium. The children who were born of the Age of Aquarius hoped that the striking of a clock would wake the gods from their slumbers to shower us with spiritual gifts. With the dawning of a new century, the freaky, fringe ideas that had become the bedrock of the New Age movement slipped effortlessly into the mainstream. Yoga, meditation, aromatherapy, angel consultations, crystal healing and anything that could be passed off as *esoteric*, or at least 'Eastern', came as close to being fashionable as it is ever likely to get. Scots, like us, raised on a diet of mince and potatoes and Calvinistic self-reliance, now can buy aromather-apy oils along with our sushi at Tesco's, the supermarket of body and soul in the New Age of Enlightenment. For those who considered themselves on a genuine spiritual quest – as opposed to simply keeping pace with celebrity wackiness – this is very bad news. However, if nothing else, this spiritual vogue shows how the rampant materialism of the West had slow-ly been found wanting.

Such spiritual disenchantment had been a long time coming, and had its most obvious genesis in the anti-materialism of the Beat generation, 50 years earlier. In his infamous poem, *Howl*, Allen Ginsberg railed against the materialism of post-war America, which was symbolized in the psy-chotic breakdown of his friend, Carl Solomon. The frustrated, enlighten-ment-seeking Everyman of Ginsberg's poem appeared driven in every conceivable enlightenment-seeking direction, all at once:

> who studied Plotinus Poe St John of the Cross telepathy and bop kabbalah because the universe instinctively vibrated at their feet in Kansas,
>
> who loned it through the streets of Idaho seeking visionary indian angels who were visionary indian angels,
>
> who thought they were only mad when Baltimore gleamed in super-natural ecstasy

Although the Beats' popularization of consciousness raising, especially when enabled by drugs, was very much a fringe event in the conservative

1950s, the practice gained critical reinforcements with the arrival of the hippie generation a decade later. By the beginning of the 21st century, illicit drug taking had almost become a convention, especially among the young, but had also (sadly) become a defence against post-modern *ennui* or apocalyptic uncertainty, rather than the key to unlock Huxley's *Doors of Perception*, or the pathway of the heart envisioned by Ginsberg and his Beat brethren.

Two hundred years ago, William Blake wrote:

> If the doors of perception were cleansed everything would appear to man as it is, infinite

In a sense, Blake provided a visual and literary language for the kind of everyday mysticism which now litters the Internet, and which has been distorted greatly by the Mirror of Interpretation. Yes, the language of spirituality has entered our vernacular, but are we any closer to embracing what the words might represent?

History may well conclude that the past 50 years of 'seeking after spiritual enlightenment' ushered in a 'New Age of Enlightenment', which made the discussion of spirituality more acceptable. This allowed people to begin to explore the deeper significance of their often all-too-mundane lives, who previously would have been excluded from the spiritual quest. In that sense, we should be thankful. However, this 'New Age' also trailed in all sorts of mud from the field of dreams of spiritual inquiry. All manner of frivolous excesses have been dragged in its wake, contributing to the dumbing down of the spiritual quest, which often has been translated into a 'McDonaldized' commodity fit for post-modern capitalism.

When we first sat down to talk about writing this book, our late friend and colleague David Brandon began his own '*Howl*' about the excesses, inaccuracies and vacuousness of much New Age spirituality. In particular, David railed against the 'mantra-chanting, incense-burning, crystal-swinging *conventionality*' of much so-called contemporary spirituality. If we remember his humorous, yet passionate, tirade correctly, it was the *mindless* conventionality that bugged him most. He was protesting at the translation of spirituality into just another piece of commercial property: spirituality born of economics – a set of tapes, a weekend retreat at a country house, our very own, ready-to-use 'course in miracles'. Any of these might bring us fulfilment, rendering us happier, turning us into 'beautiful souls', bestowing the balm of calm on our troubled lives. All promising, at least by allusion, the manna of enlightenment – at least for the small proportion of buyers who might want to go that far.

How many of those who *buy into* the commercialized spirituality that provoked David's ire is difficult to determine. The proportion is probably substantial, since much New Age spirituality appears to be merely a lever

for personal growth and is, therefore, an extension of the humanistic therapies, the 'third force' psychology that also began around the time of
Ginsberg's *Howl*. The provocative, anti-establishment, psychological
counter-culture of 'personal growth' psychology, however, has been largely assimilated into the pluralistic mainstream, hence the groaning 'self-
help' shelves in the high-street bookshops – 'happiness in 24 hours' and
'the weekend guide to enlightenment'.

Even once-arcane practices, like the Jewish *kabbalah*, which Ginsberg
jokingly called 'bop kabbalah', have become fashion accessories for the
rich and famous. *Kabbalah-lite*, as it has become known, is the latest
dream of a quick fix for the problems of living and dying. This mystical
Jewish tradition of prayer and contemplation is now becoming the latest
piece of hocus-pocus for New Age dabblers with dollars to burn. As well
as promising peace of mind, kabbalah-lite promoters offer lectures on
'What Women Want (for men only)', 'Making Love Last', 'Overcoming our
Hidden Addictions' and 'How to Read People in Five Minutes or Less'.
Obviously, the ancient mystics had a busier time than we might have
appreciated. But, as Rebecca Fowler (2003) pointed out, this pseudo-mys-
tical practice has an even more materialistic basis: promoters of kabbalah-
lite promise to arrest the ageing process, and have introduced a whole
range of kabbalah products – from mineral water, with 'wisdom in every
drop', to skincare creams to 'rejuvenate' the baggy-eyed. Kabbalah-lite
may not be making an appearance in our supermarkets for some time yet,
but, with endorsements from the likes of Madonna and Elizabeth Taylor,
it would appear to be only a matter of time.

The trivia of much New Age spiritual questing is, in our view, little more
than the commercialization of an ageless tradition. Certainly, the social
critiques and creative commentaries of the Beat and hippie generations
are important, but they merely echoed humankind's boundary-breaking,
mystical soul-searching that is, essentially, timeless. As we have travelled
the world, we have been impressed by the uniformity of traditional spiritual metaphors, and the messages that appear inherent in their often-
oblique references.

For us, spirituality has always involved our deepest feelings about life,
which link us with our past; threading through us, connecting us with the
living of life itself; emphasizing home – a sense of place in the world;
anchoring us to the land – not property, which is ephemeral – the soil that
supported our ancestors now supports us.

It did not surprise us, therefore, to find echoes of our own Celtic spirituality in the spirituality of the indigenous people of Australia, Aotearoa
(New Zealand) and North America, New World locations with very ancient
spiritual roots: places and peoples that embrace timeless connections
with the Spirit world of the past, through connection with the ground of

being in the present – the *land*. Indeed, the land provides us with another useful metaphor. The *ground* – which serves as the canvas upon which we trace the metaphorical journey of the heart; which serves as the shadow catcher for each living movement; which serves as the drum for the dancing rhythm of our footfalls – is the great servant, but also is the great teacher: yet another paradox. Our value and love of the land is bred from respect, not from an appreciation of real estate. The value of the land lies in its inherent worthlessness, which may also signal something of the paradox of the spiritual quest. We go seeking that which we already own; we pursue the gift that is already ours; we cherish the priceless truths that, essentially, are worthless.

TS Eliot, witnessed the ravages of mental distress through the experience of his first wife, Vivienne, and then spent many years in more direct confrontation with his own demons beneath the cloud of his depression. In *Little Gidding* he evoked the futile necessity of human searching:

We shall not cease from exploration
And the end of all our exploring
Will be to arrive where we started
And know the place for the first time.
Through the unknown, unremembered gate
When the last of earth left to discover
Is that which was the beginning

In our original culture, Eliot's turn for home echoes the symbolic searching embedded in Celtic knotwork, where each line threads its way outwards, as if seeking the ultimate Light, only to thread its way back to where it started. In Celtic spirituality, this starting and endpoint is the *hearth*, where the spiritual traveller will not only find warmth and comfort, but also experience, again, the Light that has always been shining (unrecognized) from within. If spirituality teaches us anything it is, as Buddha urged:

Hold to the truth within yourselves
As to the only lamp

If the appreciation of the elliptical search for the Light, through spirituality, is timeless, then its association with the field of mental health is much more recent. We have possessed a language for discussing people in mental distress, for only a few hundred years. Before the Enlightenment, everyone who defied our immediate understanding was lumped together into a swirling, tumbling lunatic mass, and was – at least to the God-fearing – evidence of demonic possession. In the 21st century, we have abandoned all such primitive explanations. Now we believe that we are more enlightened, as we play with the language of mental illness, mental disorder and (for the politically correct) mental health problems. However, this received wisdom – largely medical in origin and focus – still invokes an abstract force, which apparently takes over, and takes charge of, the person in mental distress. People may no longer be possessed by demons and other malign forces. Instead, they are *possessed* by schizophrenia or bipolar disorder – which are as invisible and malign as the demons that once possessed our fearful imaginings. It goes without saying that both are highly resistant to empirical testing. People can and do experience great distress. We appear only to have changed the names and the attributions of the 'distressors'. The science fiction film *The Invasion of the Body Snatchers*, from our 1950s' childhood, was subsequently read by film students as an allegory for the 'capture' of American minds by Communism. It could just as easily be read today as a metaphor for madness. We still do not know who or what is doing the capturing, but it certainly continues to terrify us.

Arguably, if any one thing has triggered our spiritual renaissance, it is the dehumanizing force of materialism, which reminds us to what extent we have lost touch with our deeper human values and needs, if not actually our sense of 'soul'. The scientific project first imagined by Freud aimed to kill off the ancient notion of the soul, replacing this with a more modern notion of the mind. Now, the rampant reductionism of contemporary neuroscience threatens to kill off the idea of the mind, establishing the brain not only as the medium of our experience, but also as the experience itself. *I compute therefore I am.*

Culturally, at least in the West, we have greatly over-valued physical appearances, possessions, hedonistic pleasure seeking and creature comforts, as if the acquisition and maintenance of these material 'treasures' was the point of life. Modern science approaches the problems of life and living from a similar angle, giving credence only to what can be seen and measured, believing that only the physical is *real*.

Contemporary psychiatry is typical of this materialistic world view, believing that mental illness is a function of chemical imbalance and that all so-called 'inner experience' is a mere by-product of brain activity. By focusing exclusively on the relationship between brain and behaviour, this view denies the importance of the spiritual dimensions of human nature and suggests that any such 'immeasurable' aspect of life does not *actually* exist.

Such an outlook has nurtured the crazy notion that human suffering can be eliminated, most commonly by simply popping a pill. Sadly, many of the psychotherapies, which focused on 'exploring' the experience of being human, have largely surrendered to the psychological version of this biomedical reductionism – using various psychological 'techniques' to control and contain ways of thinking and feeling. The net result is the flattening – in a normative sense – of the range of ways of being human. This is representative of the scary kinds of future-world imagined in Huxley's *Brave New World* and Orwell's *1984*. Who would have thought that the *freedom* to feel, think and believe would have represented such a threat at the beginning of the 21st century? Despite the apparent liberalization of the Western culture, the underpinning value base appears narrower than ever.

This book emphasizes the need to turn inward, listening to the various messages that are channelled through our core being. Rather than dismiss these experiences as one form of 'disorder' or another, we invite the reader to recognize the various stories that are retold here, as evidence of the difficult and often very messy soul-work, which people are often required to undertake; evidence of the spiritual quests that serendipity has organized for them; evidence of the abundant resourcefulness of the human being, when faced with the apparently 'unintelligible'. As Frattaroli (2002) recently noted, psychiatric symptoms like anxiety and depression are not themselves diseases, but are evidence of the soul's attempt to resolve an inner conflict – by forcing us to pay attention to the unconscious dark side of ourselves that we would rather ignore.

The people who have joined us, on this attempt to 'break through' the contemporary opposition to understanding the spiritual dimensions of mental health and mental distress, have struggled long and hard to gain the wisdom that informs their writing. Although the authors are not united by any specific philosophical, religious or mystical tradition, they do share an appreciation that the various struggles, which Life scatters upon the Path, have been put there for a purpose. What exactly is the purpose is not often clear, but clearing the way, surmounting the obstacles and generally taking the next, painful step appear to be what is asked of us. With each step, the point of our existence may become clearer, or it might become even more obscured. If the authors we have gathered together here are to be believed, the *outcome* is not as important as the simple fact that we have taken that next step. Knowing that we are 'on the Path' appears to be sufficient of itself.

In Part One, we consider spirituality as a reflection of the process of *change*. We provide a brief overview of the contemporary history of spiritual inquiry in the field of mental health. In Part Two, we consider spirituality as a reflection of the process of meaning-making. David Brandon cautions against any attempt to reduce spirituality to a common denominator, far less to its 'key constituents', and Ann Drysdale reminds us that the 'reality' which we experience, is – of necessity – personal. This peculiar vision of ourselves *within* our world of experience, is undoubtedly one of the building blocks of all spiritual understanding. We conclude this section with a consideration of how all our experiences – of ourselves as well as of the world outside us – are part of the *Great Whole*, the *One* that is represented by different names in all the main faith systems, but which, fundamentally, appears to be the same enduring Truth of all existence.

In Part Three, we consider spirituality in terms of different forms of *journey*. Ian Beech reviews the Buddhist appreciation of the problem of *craving*, and how our inability to ever satisfy our cravings leads to emotional pain and spiritual isolation. Liam Clarke reviews the potent power of *confession*, both as a social contract, which can weaken a person's capacity to engage in 'soul searching', and as a rich metaphor for expressing everything that we might encounter on the journey to our inner spaces. Eihblin Inglesby takes the idea of the spiritual journey one stage further by considering the traditional concept of *pilgrimage*, within which pilgrims consider not 'who' they are but 'where' they are. Sally Clay demonstrates, through her own witness, the importance of *practice* to the whole spiritual quest, and Cathy Conroy reads her own spiritual journey – in and through madness – as one imbued with *grace*. In concluding this section, Peter Wilkin reveals how we might encounter *epiphany* in everyday life, suggesting that the wisdom of the infinite lies waiting in the wings of our mundane existence.

In Part Four, we consider the potential for *healing* that lies within even the most terrifying forms of madness. Nikki Slade charts the process of disintegration and rebuilding that changed her life, and this is reviewed in a short commentary by her friend and colleague, Larry Culliford; and Sue Holt describes how the urge towards spiritual healing, which can be thrown up by madness, can often be thwarted by mental health services. Gary Platz turns the traditional role of spirituality upside-down, as he describes how his madness acted as the spur for his spiritual journey towards self-healing.

Finally, given all the references we have made here in this Preface to the quick-fix, fast-food, materialistic branding of spirituality, we conclude with a consideration of the power of 'waiting'. As many of the authors have suggested, the *practice* of life is its *purpose* and, through careful, compassionate practice, we may, ultimately, be rewarded. The critical question is not can we make the commitment, but have we the patience?

References

Eliot TS (1974) The Four Quartets. New York: Harvest Books.

Fowler R (2003) Kabbalah-lite, the cult with great skincare. The Sunday Times News Review 20 January: 5.

Frattaroli E (2002) Healing the Soul in the Age of the Brain: why medication isn't enough. New York: Penguin Putnam.

Ginsberg A (1984) Collected Poems 1947–1980. New York: Harper & Row.

Huxley A (1954) The Doors of Perception. London: Chatto and Windus.

PART ONE
Changes

Man's spiritual development is a long and arduous journey, an adventure through strange lands full of surprises, difficulties and even dangers. It involves a drastic transmutation of the 'normal' elements of the personality, an awakening of potentialities hitherto dormant, a raising of consciousness to new realms, and a functioning along a new inner dimension.

We should not be surprised. Therefore, to find that so great a change, so fundamental a transformation, is marked by several critical stages, which are not infrequently accompanied by various nervous, emotional and mental troubles.

Robert Assagioli

The song that I came to sing remains unsung to this day.
I have spent my days in stringing and unstringing my instrument.

Rabindranath Tagore

1

Spirituality and Mental Health: something for nothing?

PHIL BARKER AND POPPY BUCHANAN-BARKER

Phil Barker is a psychotherapist, academic, writer and artist. He has worked in the mental health field for almost 35 years.

> I gave up the formal world of academia recently to focus more on meaning and creativity, both of which were a dwindling currency in my professional world. Now I can work each day alongside Poppy, who has provided all sorts of inspiration to me over the years. For me, spirituality is mental health. It is largely beyond words, but can be felt, usually in the most simple of ways in the wildest of places.

Poppy Buchanan-Barker was a social worker for 26 years, working with people with a range of disabilities, and their families.

> Two years ago I established the Mental Health Recovery Consultancy – Clan Unity – with Phil. I had always worked in the 'care field', but this seemed like the right thing to do, after sharing all our hopes, dreams and disappointments throughout 36 years of marriage. We are both 'the eternal optimists' and still believe the best is yet to come. For me spirituality means many things but connection – especially being united with the past – has always been very important. Memories, of people, places and experiences, are like ribbons anchoring me to my past, while I live in the present.

Helping ourselves to a life of suffering

It may be a truism to say that life *is* suffering: we are required to undergo, experience or be subjected to various pains, losses, defeats, grief and – in particular – *change*. However, humankind still struggles to employ its

3

ingenuity to clear the world of *all* suffering. This struggle for emotional and psychological comfort is set against the blackest backdrop, as many of the world's peoples still struggle to gain daily access to clean water, and vast numbers live on the edges of the precipices of war, famine and pestilence. Even as Western scientists claim to have unravelled the mystery of human life – to be on the brink of a 'theory of everything' – those ancient bogeys, the Four Horsemen of the Apocalypse, still ride roughshod over much of the earth.

As we prepared the final draft of this book, the media was ablaze with the story that the Raelian 'cult' had stolen a march on the world's top scientists by cloning the first human child. It would have been bad enough if the perpetrators of what many saw as the 'reckless abandonment of the rigour of science' had been mere rogue biologists, focused perhaps on making money from the emergent cloning technology. The possibility, however, that science might have been overtaken by someone in the pay of an 'extremist cult' caused much pompous posturing about the near-sanctity of science, and the need for control over the use of science's progeny, *technology*.

Perhaps this great brouhaha betrayed the deep nature of our shared anxieties concerning fiddling with the life force. If the evidence for cloning is examined carefully, the possibility of reproducing exact replicas of any species, far less replicas of our dead pets or children, is as far off as ever. The dream of pop genetics doesn't quite match the reality.

In effect, the Raelians trumped the excessive optimism of the whole human genome mapping programme with their highly public, unsubstantiated claims about cloning. They knew how to seduce a media hungry for more evidence of humankind's capacity to match, if not triumph over, the forces of nature. Indeed, our hunger for improving our lot, or at least the lot of those with the money to pay, is one of the hallmarks of the age. In the context of the spiritual life – whether Taoist or Christian, Muslim or New Age – this hunger is insatiable. The more we try to feed it, the hungrier it becomes.

Arguably, the other great deception of our post-modern age is the much-vaunted notion of self-help, which has much in common with the human building and repairing programme dreamed of by the biotechnologists. When the Scotsman Samuel Smiles first promoted the idea of self-improvement more than a hundred years ago, he would never have dreamed that it would grow into one of the juggernauts of the New Age. Ironically, Smiles believed that:

> Practical wisdom is only to be learned in the school of experience. Precepts and instruction are useful so far as they go, but, without the discipline of real life, they remain of the nature of theory only.

Today, the self-help book is the short cut to the search for fulfilment, growth and personal development that was anathema to Smiles, who saw, in all the 'great men' of his day, the virtuous evidence of thrift, duty and character. Although Smiles did not suggest that it was necessary to *suffer* to grow as a person, he recognized the value of failure and hardship as setting conditions for negotiating change. Today's self-help movement has other ideas.

In his ironic novel, the Canadian writer Will Ferguson (2002) poked fun at the self-help book and the publishing industry that feeds from it. In *Happiness*™, his fictional publisher launches the self-help book to end all self-help books. When published, calamity ensues because *Happiness*™ – unlike all other self-help books – actually delivers on its promises. As readers lose weight, stop smoking, enjoy otherworldly sex and discover True Happiness, chaos overtakes America, which experiences an 'apocalyptic plague of happiness', collapsing the economy in a benign pile of self-satisfaction. Only a comic novel – or an allegory for the hunger pangs of the New Age of Enlightenment?

The ambitions of medical technology and the fast-feeding side of the self-help movement raise questions about the value of suffering. The traditional belief that suffering might be beneficial, at least in small doses, has largely been overtaken by the assumption that pain of any kind is to be tranquillized, anaesthetized or avoided altogether. The original Latin root suggests that suffering involves the 'bearing' of something arduous. Not surprisingly, we talk of people of upright or stoical bearing and, especially in the Christian tradition, associate bearing with the cross: a symbol, perhaps, for all humankind's suffering. These linguistic roots are also to be found in the concept of the 'patient',[1] who is required to tolerate, endure or *suffer*, physically, mentally or both. However, with the rise of various psychiatric 'survivor' and 'consumer' movements around the world, people who have been required to endure 'mental illness' and treatment for their 'illness', have distanced themselves from the traditional labels of medicine. Consequently, the concept of *patient*-hood has acquired pejorative associations. The possible significance of psychic suffering has been obscured by a barrage of alternative, often politically correct euphemisms.[2]

---

[1] (L) *patiens, patientis*: present participle of *pati*, to suffer.

[2] Where people once were defined *by professionals* as 'schizophrenics' or 'psychotic patients', many people now *define themselves* as 'people with a serious or enduring mental illness', or more simply, 'users' or 'consumers' (of mental health services). One way or another, both kinds of descriptors suggest that the often short-term, and certainly never *constant*, experience of psychic disturbance defines the person. We would rather take the view that the subject in question is a *person*, first and foremost, who sometimes is like this (e.g. happy), and at other times is like that (e.g. sad). Unfortunately, this implies that such persons are more like the rest of us than different. Such egalitarianism appears to be too radical even for the 21st century.

Perhaps our vain ambitions to avoid suffering, or at least not to name it as such, merely generate more suffering. Although we take no pleasure in pain – whether physical or emotional – we recognize, at least in the light of our own experience, that lessons can be learned. Experience – especially when facilitated by Mistress Unreason – can be a harsh teacher.

All alone: fear, losing and loathing

Psychic suffering takes many forms, especially when we talk of psychological problems, mental illness or plain old-fashioned madness. Threaded through much human distress is the ancient and pervasive spectre of *fear*. Meditating on the grief he felt after his wife's death CS Lewis (1961) observed:

> No one ever told me that grief felt so like fear. I am not afraid, but the sensation is like being afraid. The same fluttering in the stomach, the same restlessness, the yawning. I keep on swallowing.

The experience of loss reminds us that the final threat we face is our ultimate *aloneness*. In *The Rime of the Ancient Mariner*, Coleridge offered a metaphor for humankind's blind rejection of everything that lies beyond our existing knowledge. Anything not already part of our received wisdom is to be feared and, if possible, controlled. By killing the albatross, the mariner was forced to face the emptiness of his isolated existence:

> Alone, alone, all, all alone,
> Alone on a wide wide sea!
> And never a saint took pity on
> My soul in agony.

Only with time, and the wisdom of hindsight, does the now *ancient* mariner come to understand the meaning of his once bloody act:

> He prayeth well, who loveth well
> Both man and bird and beast.
> He prayeth best, who loveth best
> All things both great and small.

Coleridge's poetry and philosophical writing was shot through with self-doubt and a metaphysical anxiety that anticipated modern existentialism. Although hardly a spiritual text, Coleridge's poem carries some important messages about experience, fear, responsibility and humankind's almost insignificant scale on the wider canvas of existence.

So, what are we most afraid of knowing? Although we learn about death, often from an early age, the experience of our own mortality can be quite different. The recognition that, ultimately, we are insignificant, at least in the wider sphere of things, if not in the cosmic sense, is a terrifying insight. If we are only 'here' for such a short time – cosmically speaking – what is the point? Indeed, physicists often argue that because the universe is finite, and ultimately will self-destruct, there is no point to our existence. Although this is not going to happen tomorrow, even in cosmological terms, such a scientific insight sends many people scurrying in search of 'other worldly salvation', perhaps even like the Raelians, in the prospect of rescuers from a parallel universe.

For those of us who settle for life on earth, many spend our lives trying to find ourselves in others, seeking shelter in their shade, only – like Lewis – to risk losing that shelter, revealing, violently, the scale of our aloneness. Although the pain of such suffering is necessary, it may not be the endpoint of suffering. It may only be a staging post. Our suffering – whether of the grief of melancholy or the grief of loss – may only be signalling the way to an even more significant destination. As the Buddha suggested (Goddard, 1956):

> Be ye lamps unto yourselves.
> Be your own reliance.
> Hold to the truth within yourselves
> As to the only lamp.

But what is this 'truth' for which we search? And how do we know that we are on the right path, however brightly lit? Why do we find the experience of loss – whether of our kith and kin, or simply 'loss of control' – so loathsome?

The reader will not be surprised to hear that we believe this to be a function of the spiritual vacuum of contemporary life. Once our losses were borne (suffered/endured) with some serenity – whether we were peasants or kings. This may not have helped to promote health, since health is never a function of any one specific aspect of our lives, but, for at least the past 20 years, we have recognized the dangers of this 'spiritual vacuum' for healthcare. At the Assembly of the World Health Organization in 1983, Al-Awadi (1983) appealed for a wider appreciation of the role of the spiritual in the construction of health:

> material progress in the present world has reached levels unprecedented in past history or civilisation. Yet we find that what prevails in this world are anxiety and apprehension, so much so that one could say that the distinguishing feature of this age is a sense of loss and uncertainty. We have stripped man, over the last decades, of his spiritual values, and materialism is now in full control of all aspects of our life to the extent that man feels lost and restless, desperately seeking tranquillity and peace of mind ... I am quite certain that regardless of what we do to provide health care for the

body and the mind, man shall remain lost and restless until we provide for the spiritual aspects of life.

Evidently, the call to spiritual re-armament is no recent phenomenon.

Psychiatry and the soul

At least in principle, psychiatry sought to study the soul, although many of those who cast themselves as 'psychiatric survivors' might be forgiven for laughing aloud at this historical relic (Newnes et al., 2000). The Hellenistic personification of the soul (*psyche*) was sometimes represented visually as a butterfly, evoking its fragility, beauty and movement; and most English dictionaries acknowledge that *psyche* means soul and spirit first, with mind a latter day understanding. This betrays the original Greek root *psukhé*, which meant breath, life and *soul*. Regrettably, the soul has fallen through the floor of mainstream psychiatry, although a tiny number of psychiatrists are trying to reinstate this ancient focus (Culliford, 2002).

The psychotherapeutic arm of psychiatry has followed, perhaps unwittingly, the path recommended by the Buddha and Socrates, who both suggested the power of 'looking within', examining life as a way of finding meaning. Indeed, understanding of life and our part *of* it, and *in* it, may be both the beginning and end of the spiritual journey that often begins in psychotherapy, but cannot be completed in such an ultimately *mundane* activity.

However, the traditional therapeutic processes seem able only to offer transitory relief from the emptiness and alienation felt by people caught up in the spiritual crisis, which is embedded in certain forms of madness. As Karasu (1999) observed, they are so limited because, in general, mainstream forms of psychotherapy (and psychiatric treatment) address *individual pathology* rather than the wider aspects of human being.

The person who is caught in the spiral of madness is trying, desperately, to return to wholeness – feeling as if they are threatened with complete disintegration. For many, this begins with self-realization and the search for meaning, exploring as LeShan (1999) has observed, the states of being that appear to use the most of themselves. Traditional psychiatry and psychotherapy use, instead, a historical-pathological approach, trying to establish how the person 'became' like this. We should, perhaps, be exploring what this whole process of collapse and disintegration might be about, and especially what might be its hidden meanings, if not what the person might be trying to accomplish within the spiritual crisis.

In pursuit of such unashamedly 'spiritual' aims, therapists need to move themselves from believing in 'fixing' psychopathology, towards believing in the person's capacity for transformation. In Karasu's view, the subject of therapy is not a *patient* or a *client* (far less a 'user' or 'consumer') but 'an uninitiated human being' (Karasu, 1999). Rather than employing specific 'techniques' of therapy, therapists must be open to whatever works, especially 'being with the other', which targets the spiritual centre. Karasu is – arguably – the leading voice for the spiritual transformation of psychotherapy to have emerged from mainstream psychiatry.

By emphasizing his belief that what *really matters* is not the particular school of psychotherapy, but the openness, humility and even ignorance of the therapist, Karasu (2001) has challenged the traditional professional empire of psychotherapy and psychiatry. In his most recent work, Karasu (2003) has acknowledged that material possessions, success, power and pleasure often fail to fill the void that lies at the heart of our lives. Getting married and divorced, taking drugs and engaging in other 'high-risk' activities may result in a temporary abatement of our spiritual unease. For many, the life of a 'spiritual tourist' (Brown, 1998) may offer some reassurance but, ultimately, the hollow feeling that 'something is missing' returns. As far as Karasu is concerned, we have no option but to begin to explore the deepest yearnings of our heart. Especially in the West, our greatest yearning may be for 'happiness' (Pepper, 1992; Whiteside, 2001), but as Karasu notes, there is no end to the journey to 'real happiness'. Indeed, there is not even a good place to start. Karasu urges us to start *here*, where we are, to begin the journey NOW! This echoes the traditional Tibetan Buddhist emphasis on *embracing* rather than denying the painful aspects of our lives (Chödrön, 1994). The fear of loss – especially of our 'sanity' and selfhood – may lie at the very heart of the spiritual vacuum of our lives, and may even deter us from taking that first, necessary step into the next moment.

Spirituality and mental health

If we forget about the centuries-long association between madness and demonic possession, spirituality and mental health have enjoyed only brief flirtations. Only time will tell whether this will turn into a meaningful relationship. The reference to demons reminds us that religion represents a special class of spiritual experience. Especially within the Christian tradition, evil spirits have been represented as a virtual plague on the houses of people who came to be classed as 'mentally ill'. Oftentimes the person so 'possessed' was seen as deserving of such a hellish intrusion. Sinful ways and a general wandering from the path of righteousness brought people into contact with the demon, who clutched at their very soul. This tradition offers, however, only a limited frame of reference for what we understand as 'the spiritual'. Clearly, there is a difference between religion and spirituality, if only because some practitioners of religion, and the bureaucracy of the faith they profess, often appear bereft of any spiritual quality. History suggests that religion often becomes merely a crutch for living with worldly trials and tribulations, or a lever for manipulating adherence to rules and conventions, which are transparently social or cultural. The location of the Godhead in our lives, and humankind's meaningful place in the wider, cosmic reading of our relationship to the Spiritual Other, are often religiously indistinct. More often it is obscured by the internecine disputes that have ravaged most organized religions.

Does the world of spirituality fare any better? Does 'spirituality' offer a clear, less ambiguous message as to what it might all be, ultimately, about? To be concrete for a moment, all readers will be 'believers', either in one religion or faith system or another (or perhaps several), *or* they will be agnostics, atheists or 'rationalists' – their core belief is in being an 'unbeliever'. However, they will all believe in something, if only that the universe is ultimately meaningless and that we are simply adding personal and social footnotes to Darwinian evolution. The 'spiritually inclined' among us are drawn from both of these faith camps. Some of the seekers, those who have tired of traditional faith systems' inability to deliver whatever it is they were looking for, may be drawn to the world of 'spirituality'. A similar trek may be made out of the land of reason, by those who – having rejected all religious thought – are still asking: 'Surely there must be more to it than this?' Will these seekers find what they are looking for? What exactly are they looking for? Eternal life or salvation? Forgiveness for a misspent life or a return to the comfort of the Father (or Mother) of all Creation?

The yearning for a sense of the sacred, especially when pursued avidly by affluent Westerners, can often appear foolhardy. Mick Brown (1998) illustrated vividly how the spiritual quest had become a leitmotif of 20th-century life. The 'road less travelled' by the spiritual tourist encompasses the holy and the lost, the wise and the foolish, all journeying inwards in search of illumination.

The lemming-like rush for such illumination was captured by Rachel Storm (1991) in her excellent exposé of the history and development of the New Age. While much of the spiritual yearning that she uncovered seemed pathetic, if not adolescent, she recognized that the wisdom people sought might well be 'out there'. 'Where' they might find it, was never clarified. She concluded with a pithy quotation from a Rajneesh sannyasin:

> The danger of the New Age is that amidst all the spiritual slogans that sound
> like truth there are actually a few pearls of wisdom. But for that one real

mystic rose there are ninety-nine plastic look-alikes that cost less, last longer and promise instant enlightenment.

The real pilgrimage to truth takes guts, integrity and putting your whole life at stake – the New Age variety takes Visa, Mastercard and putting aside three minutes a day chanting under a pyramid tepee for lower interest rates. All in all ... people aren't actually interested in the 'real' ...

Storm (1991: 207)

Culliford (2002: 251) cited research that suggested that a:

Survey of 200 London psychiatrists found that 90% viewed religious beliefs as relevant to patient mental health 'to be considered during assessment and therapy'.

He also noted the 'official advice' of the Royal College of Psychiatrists (2000: 41), that:

Good practice in general adult psychiatry will include: taking a direct care role which involves assessment of mental health problems ... and being cognisant of the *spiritual* and cultural needs of patients and their carers ... understanding and referring appropriately in respect of social, *spiritual* or cultural interventions [emphases added].

Such leadership is obviously welcome, although many 'survivors' might question how such *cognisance* of their spiritual needs is translated into action. Many users of 'mental health' services have described abysmal standards of care, especially in psychiatric units in London, where even respect and dignity appeared to receive little attention, far less the cognisance of, and response to, spiritual needs (e.g. Rose, 2000). We would not expect established authorities like the Royal College of Psychiatrists – or their international equivalents – to deny the perceived importance of the spiritual impulse. Changing the psychiatric method to express respect for its actual importance may well be another thing. Perhaps, however, we need to clarify what is meant by 'mental health' before we can explore how the spiritual might be addressed.

Mental health and meaning

In Australia, the Queensland Health Authority defined mental health as:

A dynamic process in which a person's physical, cognitive, affective, behavioural and social dimensions interact functionally with one another and with the environment.

In the USA the Surgeon General (US Department of Health and Human Services, 1999) defined it as referring to:

> ... the successful performance of mental function, resulting in productive activities, fulfilling relationships with other people, and the ability to adapt to change and cope with adversity.

Both definitions betray an emphasis on *function* and *efficacy*, making it clear that anyone who is not *productively* engaged, or who experiences *unfulfilling* relationships or even the occasional flutter of disquiet in the face of everyday challenges, is *not* mentally healthy. As with all such bureaucratic definitions of health and wellbeing, one is left wondering who does fit these stringent criteria.

One thing is clear even if we found it difficult to classify a person with a discrete mental *illness*, it would not be difficult to define that individual as mentally *unhealthy*. The future of 'mental health services' seems, therefore, to be safely assured, whatever they actually do by way of promoting and enabling 'mental health' in practice.

Perhaps because of the problems of adequately defining mental health, the past decade has witnessed a switch of emphasis to the facilitation of recovery, which Anthony (1993) defined as:

> ... a deeply personal, unique process of changing one's attitudes, values, feelings, goals, skills and/or roles. It is a way of living a satisfying, hopeful, and contributing life even with limitations caused by the illness. Recovery involves the development of new meaning and purpose in one's life as one grows beyond the catastrophic effects of mental illness.

The emphasis on growing through and beyond the experience of distress, and especially the focus on *meaning*, seems to redefine the mental health agenda, bringing it closer to a consideration of the 'point' of a person's life. Such a *point* might involve not only questing for meaning in life, but also – as Frankl (2000) has argued – begging the 'question whether any such meaning exists at all'. Certainly, this meaningful emphasis – from the writings of people like Patrica Deegan (1996) in the USA, to Julie Leibrich in New Zealand – shifts our focus beyond the internal functioning alluded to in most bureaucratic definitions of mental health, to an appreciation of the almost ineffable, emergent story of the person's life (Leibrich, 1999).

For Leibrich, meaning is always *there* – in the story of our lives – whether we are aware of it or not. The journey of recovery may be no more than the long walk to recognition of that meaning. For us, the journey is often taken on uncharted seas, invoking the dangers of the deep as well as of distance (Barker, 2002). Leibrich (1999) sees the story as a gift, even when it involves the pain of madness:

The act of telling stories can restore people ('re-store'). The telling of our story to someone who is genuinely interested and who relates to the telling through their own experiences is a very precious thing (p. 5).

In a very real sense the story makes its own journey in search of greater understanding, which can be found in the true listener. This explains in some way why people 'talk to God' and often claim to have been 'heard' (O'Brien, 1964).

Leibrich's appreciation for the story-journey is illustrated by reference to Janet Frame:

But if a story is told and not understood, then a part of oneself has reached out into nothingness.
They died because the words they had spoken
Returned always homeless to them[3]
Some people even say when you lose your story, you lose yourself (p. 6).

This sense of communication is echoed in most commonly accepted definitions of spirituality, which is often understood to involve some kind of a partnership with one's Higher Power or Godhead, with Nature or with the Absolute. As Culliford (2002) noted, spirituality can provide hope and solace during the person's crisis or experience of illness. Individually, this might take the form of a sense of peace and, within group settings, a sense of understanding and social support.

Although often projected as being 'unworldly', the engagement with the spiritual life is a highly practical and grounded activity. Evelyn Underhill (1937) reminded us that:

Our favourite distinction between the spiritual life and practical life is false. We cannot divide them ... For a spiritual life is simply a life in which all that we do comes from the centre, where we are anchored in God: a life soaked through and through by a sense of His reality and claim, and self-given to the great movement of His will.

In that sense, spirituality is more of an essential than a luxury, where people eventually realize that they have no choice but to be on the spiritual path:

It was what people kept telling me. I felt as I always did at such times, stranded between reason and a craving for faith, uncomfortable in the knowledge that while a spiritual belief may lead you to believe in anything, a materialist outlook on life will lead you to believe nothing.

(Brown, 1998: 290)

---

[3] From 'The Suicides'. In *The Pocket Mirror* by Janet Frame, Vintage, 1992.

The Celtic perspective

However, talking about spirituality, other than in vague terms, is well nigh impossible. We fumble with metaphors, attempting to evoke an appreciation of the experience, which lies beyond words. As St Augustine said: 'If you don't ask me, I know; if you ask me, I don't know!' (Montgomery, 1910). We all have a sense of what we mean by the word but have a hard time clearly defining it. We attempt to answer this question with our heads while spirituality is primarily a matter of our hearts. For us, spirituality is a question without an answer: something we look for but do not actually expect to find. As we try to live our lives in pursuit of a higher understanding of ourselves, God and the Universe, we examine all that we know of what is inside and outside of ourselves.

In the Celtic tradition of spirituality, the journey we take *towards* understanding always leads home. John O'Donohue (1997) reminds us that, although we are often told that the spiritual journey involves a sequence of stages, this is an illusion:

> When time is reduced to linear progress it is emptied of presence. Meister Eckhart ... says that there is no such thing as a spiritual journey ... if there were a spiritual journey, it would be only a quarter-inch long, though many miles deep. It would be a swerve into rhythm with your deeper nature and presence ... You do not need to go away outside your self to come into real conversation with your soul and the mysteries of your spiritual world. *The eternal is at home* – within you (p. 120, emphasis added).

Despite being at the other side of the world, Julie Leibrich found a similar understanding:

> It is a kind of coming home. For me, the meaning of spirituality is meaning itself (Leibrich, 2001).

Liebrich's experience may well be signalling an important 'change of heart' in the whole field of spirituality and mental health:

> My definition of mental health has a lot in common with the way I define spirituality. Both concepts are concerned with the experience of self. One reaching into dimensions of space to discover self, the other realising the freedom that comes from accepting self. That is why spiritual experiences and their interpretation can have such a profound influence on mental health.

Leibrich's appreciation that there might be something 'in' the space of her Self that might ultimately be of great value echoes an ancient story told by John O'Donohue (1997).

As a mark of respect, an old man brought melons every day to his king who, not wanting to insult the man, accepted them graciously, then tossed them into his back garden. One evening, just as the old man was about to hand over the melon, a monkey jumped down and knocked the melon from his hand, shattering it on the ground, sending a shower of diamonds from its heart. When the king went into his garden, he found that all the other melons had melted away, leaving a hillock of precious jewels.

O'Donohue notes:

The moral of this story is that sometimes in awkward situations, in problems or in difficulties, all that is awkward is the disguise. Very often at the heart of the difficulty, there is the light of a great jewel. It is wise to embrace with hospitality that which is awkward and difficult (p. 197).

Some people who have been in states of extreme madness have come to appreciate the disguise of their distress and the great insights that lie nestled in its heart (Barker et al., 1999).

The paradox of individualism

Short or long, deep or shallow, the spiritual trek is taken alone. Yet, the individual occupies a curious and critical place in the whole process of *being* and *becoming*. Clearly, we all face suffering alone, even when that is inflicted on the group, if not a whole people, as in 'ethnic cleansing' (Frankl, 2000). All experience is individual, but suffering often hammers home the isolated nature of the endurance of reality. Perhaps because the success of society is so dependent on aggregating human experience, *normalizing* it, those who seek individual paths of self-discovery are destined to come into conflict with 'social truths', which derive from statistical representations of 'normality'.

Psychology and psychiatry represent grand narratives of what it *means* to be human. These are expressed as various theories of the human condition. They cancel out individual experience in favour of rules that appear to apply to the majority. Ironically, these general theories apply to no one in particular. As Jung (1961) observed:

Any theory formulates an *ideal average* which abolishes all exceptions at either end of the scale and replaces them by an abstract mean. This mean is quite valid, though it need not necessarily occur in reality ... If I determine the weight of each stone in a bed of pebbles and get an average weight of 145 grams, this tells me very little about the real nature of pebbles ... This is particularly true of theories which are based on statistics. The distinctive thing about real facts, however, is their individuality. Not to put too fine a point on it, one could say that the real picture consists of nothing but exceptions to the rule, and that, in consequence, absolute reality has predominantly the character of *irregularity*.

Most people are aware of their own *uniqueness* and 'irregularity', if only intuitively, but are convinced, by the power of psychology (and more recently the media), that their individuality is somehow less *real* than some generalized theory about people and the human condition. As these 'general rules' of humanity – derived from psychology, sociology and psychiatry – have increasingly taken hold in the social consciousness, the individual is, correspondingly, deprived of the moral decision as to how he or she should live life (Szasz, 1996). When 'the person' asks questions *of* 'the person' *about* the nature of *being* that person, a personal theory of being and becoming emerges. Alan Watts (1977) was aware of the paradoxes such self-inquiry involved:

> So long as I identify myself with my conscious intention, and voluntary mind, I feel that I am in control of relatively few events. But I realise that this identification is after all a matter of opinion, of social convention, of an acquired way of describing myself to myself. Both Buddhist and Hindu disciplines of spiritual growth (i.e. meditation or yoga) consist primarily of exploring the question 'what am I?'
>
> (Watts, 1977: 117)

Today, neuroscience is the latest 'grand theory' of the human condition to emerge. It explains what it is to *be* and *feel* human, as a function of neurochemical events in the brain. In psychology – and to some extent psychotherapy – the superficial pragmatism of cognitive psychology is in its ascendancy. Not all practitioners of the dominant mode of therapy – *cognitive behaviour therapy* (CBT) – deny the possible spiritual nature and meanings of extreme states, such as psychosis. However, those who are more reductively inclined often try to guide the person towards a 're-adjustment to the dominant paradigm (insight) at the cost of the individual journey' (Clarke, 2002). This may be socially helpful but spiritually disastrous.

The great paradox of human experience is that, when restrained from appreciating this individuality and uniqueness, the person can experience a loss of a sense of 'self'. However, when life is devoted, wholly, to the pursuit of 'selfhood' – as in hedonism – a similar loss of selfhood can emerge. *How* people confront and explore their individuality, and the *purpose* of such self-seeking, seems more important.

The futility of explanation

Many of the grand psychological theories of the human condition appear to diminish (or reduce to absurdity) the complex issues involved in being and becoming human. Increasingly, we classify and categorize all human functioning in the language of psychiatry. All *distress* is a function of some dysfunction worthy of treatment. All *evil* is a function of some personality disorder, even if impossible to 'treat'. In Jung's view humankind's trust in *reason* had produced a fragmentation of our realities: especially the unreasonable splitting of the world into 'good and evil', 'saints and sinners'. In Jung's view, everyone carried the 'shadow' within their psyche, and merely tried to project it into other groups (like communists) or individuals (psychopaths). Regrettably, one outcome of this 'splitting' is that we fail to acknowledge our inherent weaknesses, which are essential aspects of *who* we are and *what* we might become.

Neuroscientists risk reducing the experience of being human to truly absurd proportions, by trying to explain all human experience in neurochemical terms. Francis Crick, for example, recently claimed that ultimately we would be able to demonstrate that:

> You, your joys and your sorrows, your memories and your ambitions, your sense of personal identity and free will, are in fact no more than the behaviour of a vast assembly of nerve cells and their associated molecules.
>
> (Crick, 1995: 3)

Crick believed that his approach to the mind reflected a new idea but, as Szasz (1996) noted, this was because he was ignorant of the history of the mind and especially of madness. Notably, Crick insisted that his approach to the problem of the mind was scientific but this was:

> a claim he supports by denying agency to persons and attributing agency to things. In Crick's world, neural networks 'learn' and free will (capitalized) is an attribute of the cerebral cortex. He asks: 'Where might Free Will be located in the brain?' and answers: 'Free Will is located in or near the anterior cingulated sulcus'.
>
> (Szasz, 1996: 84)

We would despair if such profound experiences as 'despair' were not defined, largely, as epiphenomenal to the core brain function of 'us'. Thankfully, Szasz's gentle irony is a valuable antidepressant.

The neuroscientific discourse is vital to our consideration of madness and spirituality. People in the grip of madness are entrapped in a consideration of self-hood that many of us avoid by throwing ourselves into various 'normalizing' activities. Madness often involves the perennial existential crisis: who am I and what, on earth, am I doing here? This is not to say that other critical phenomena are not involved in the construction of this human crisis – signposts, en route to the ultimate concerns the person will express about her or his 'selfhood'. However, the *core* crisis, if such a metaphor is not inappropriate, involves the person's presumed relationship with Self, albeit by dint of some troublesome relations with the Other.

Elio Frattaroli believes that contemporary psychiatry is in imminent danger of losing its mind. Instead of treating patients as mere chemical configurations, Frattaroli proposes that we should learn to recognize and find compassion for the feelings that inform our lives. Only by dealing with our selves and our souls can we ever create true healing.

Given his evident feelings of unease with the medical model of psychiatry, which holds that emotions stem from brain chemistry, which can readily be altered through drugs, Frattaroli's argument could be read as anti-psychiatric. It might be better to recognize his *pro-human* emphasis. When we hypothesize that anxiety, shame and guilt, for example, are meaningless neurological glitches, rather than urgent calls to self-reflection, we promote the pharmacological quick fix, at the expense of attending to the deeper, long-term needs of the soul.

No guru, no method, no teacher

So, how do we respond to extreme forms of human distress? It has been estimated that there are, literally, several hundred forms of 'therapy'. These variants of psychoanalysis, counselling and behaviour therapy try to find simpler or more efficient ways to 'fix' various forms of human distress. When we consider what human distress might 'mean' – in spiritual terms – the wisdom of 'fixing', as opposed to developing understanding, might be questioned. Indeed, many people make discoveries *within* psychotherapy, which appear to have little to do with the therapeutic method, or even the therapist, but may be a function of their own reflection: no more and no less (Barker and Kerr, 2000; Karasu, 2001). In that sense, the therapist – and the therapeutic method – may only be providing a *context*, or setting, for the person to engage in a necessary act of reflecting (Barker and Kerr, 2000).

In this consumerist age, many therapists now sell their wares on television, marketing themselves and their 'new' methods as the answer to all manner of human ills. The influence of the grand theories of human experience, which originally deprived people of their individuality – and their individual morality – helps in this selling process, whereby psyches are shaped and modified by presenters on daytime television. The idea that these therapies (and their sophisticated therapists) are unnecessary is a threatening concept. If the Emperor really has no 'new clothes', then people must confront their own individuality and make their own choices, if not their own 'clothes', as they reflect on their own experience, coming to their own realization of who they are and what is the ultimate meaning of their lives (Frankl, 2000).

Meditation in life

The reflection, which is a necessary part of some forms of psychotherapy, is akin to meditation. When people appreciate that reflection is the *beginning*, *middle* and *end* of the therapeutic endeavour, then therapy becomes a spiritual undertaking (Karasu, 1999). The reflection process helps the person to appreciate that *who* he or she is, is a function of *how* he or she lives. The understanding of living emerges from the experience of doing. Reading spiritual works may make one *wiser*, but meditation makes one *better*. Where the person allows the 'silent conversation' its fullest rein, then it can become a silent conversation with God (however defined), within which may be revealed the meaning not just of distress but of life itself.

Living *and* doing: living *as* doing

The experience of reflecting – specifically – on life problems (the common focus of therapy) is easily extended, through meditation, to the reflection on the essence of life itself. Such reflection need not be complex, and certainly does not require complex training or sophisticated techniques. Indeed, there are as many 'meditation merchants' as there are psychotherapy salespeople. Those who would try to turn it into a 'product' often obscure the simplicity of meditation and its many potential rewards. As Marcus Aurelius observed:

> Nowhere does a man retire with more quiet or freedom than into his own soul.

The inherent emptiness of meditation is often sufficient to allow us to confront the futility of post-modern life, with all its striving and struggling, helping us to appreciate more clearly the purpose of life and one's ultimate destiny. Wallace (1989) believed that even simple forms of meditation provide access to an intelligence that transcends even the most sophisticated forms of education:

> It is quite possible that in all your years of education, you have never been trained to cultivate the simple form of quiescent, stable, lucid awareness. If so, you probably found that much of that five minute period [in meditation] was spent in conceptual distraction, and even when the attention was on the breath it lacked clarity and continuity. Such an undisciplined mind is a poor instrument for empirically investigating the nature of cognitive or physical events. This unrefined state of consciousness also makes us prone to unnecessary suffering when the mind is dominated by such emotions as fear, resentment, guilt and aggression (p. 168).

Arguably, the most prevalent human problem of the day is 'low self-esteem'. Paradoxically, as people meditate on their own, essential, unimportance – in the cosmic sense – their inherent value grows. Meditation allows the person to develop a buffer against the tongues of both flatterers and critics, eradicating the itch for praise, allowing our natural, inherent light to illuminate us from *within*.

Returning to the absolute

It is by no means necessary, or even desirable, to try to construe therapy in spiritual terms. However, the threats present in an increasingly material culture appear to be bringing more and more people, perhaps unwittingly, to an appreciation of the emptiness of their lives, and the need to see beyond themselves, into the infinite. As people look into the reflection of themselves and the construction of their own lives, they may gain a glimpse of the Absolute that serves as the backdrop to their human struggles. As CS Lewis (1961) remarked:

> Of course it's easy enough to say that God seems absent at our greatest need because He is absent – non-existent. But then why does He seem so present when, to put it quite frankly, we don't ask for Him?

Indeed, the realization of our own individual importance – and yet, at the same time unimportance – may be an essential part of the continued development of humanity. As Jung noted:

> It is, unfortunately, only too clear that if the individual is not truly regenerated, society cannot be either. (Instead of roping the individual into a social organisation, reducing him to a condition of diminished responsibility, the Churches should) be raising him out of the torpid, mindless mass and making it clear to him that he is the one important factor and that the salvation of the world consists in the salvation of the individual soul.

Wrestling with the angel, on very thin ice

Although presently fashionable, the contemporary pairing of spirituality and mental health may, in years to come, provoke much head scratching. Certainly, the contemporary critic of such a development might well argue that many (if not most) people in states of high anxiety, deep despair or extreme alienation – whether from self or others – are *disturbed*, and that this disturbance lies somewhere, or perhaps in several places, within the physical body. In that sense, not much has changed since Hippocrates' day. However, it could also be said that any 'disturbing' experience shields the potential for spiritual revelation. There is no logical reason why people described as 'mentally ill' should be excluded from such revelations. As many of the authors gathered together in this book show, education, socialization and plain old-fashioned 'trying too hard' to gain enlightenment may represent barriers to the experience of the spiritual.

What is the difference between the tortured soul of Coleridge's *Ancient Mariner* and the tortured experiences of those who have encountered what has been called madness and now, patronisingly, is referred to as *mental health problems*? Political correctness demands that any experience, which anyone wishes to *call* spiritual, must be accepted as such. But this is the terrorism of acceptance, which can be just as imposing as the terrorism of rejection.

We would urge caution against simply accepting, at face value, any unusual experience as evidence of an encounter with the Absolute, however we might wish to define this. Equally, we would urge caution against the simplistic distinction between 'spiritual emergence' and plain old-fashioned madness. When the New Zealand writer Janet Frame was given a diagnosis of schizophrenia, this led to years of futile and damaging psychiatric treatment. As her biographer suggested, the writer, who had experienced a huge number of emotional and spiritual upheavals in her early life, was 'wrestling with the angel' (King, 2001). Arguably, she was in the eye of the storm of spiritual emergence and should never have been diagnosed as mentally ill, far less institutionalized. However, Sally Clay (1999) was, by her own admission, possessed by madness, yet she too was like Jacob, wrestling with the angel. And so she wrote:

> Jacob named the place of his struggle Peniel, which means 'face of God'. I too have seen God face to face, and I want to remember my Peniel. I really do not want to be called recovered. From the experience of madness I received a wound that changed my life. It enabled me to help others and to know myself. I am proud that I have struggled with God and with the mental health system.
>
> I have not recovered. I have overcome (p. 15).

We have spent a sum total of 60 years working with people in varying states of madness, social estrangement and spiritual flux. We have also encountered some of these states, face to face. Although we can recognize *when* people are in a state of madness, or are estranged from themselves or others, or are 'wrestling with the angel', we are hesitant about providing any formula for discriminating such states, for often they clearly overlap, if not – as in Sally Clay's case – belong, each to the other.

Ultimately, this book is a journey taken across perilously thin ice and the steps taken are tentative. If the reader hears the authors exclaim '*ah-*

ba', these are just as likely to arise from the experience of slipping and floundering as from any genuine revelation. We can live with such uncertainty. We hope that the reader will be similarly philosophical.

References

Al-Awadi ARA (1983) The delegates speak. WHO Chronicle 37: 131.

Anthony WA (1993) Recovery from mental illness: the guiding vision of the mental health service system in the 1990s. Innovations & Research 2: 17–24.

Aurelius M (1964) Marcus Aurelius: meditations (translated by M Staniforth). London: Penguin.

Barker P (2002) The Tidal Model: the healing potential of metaphor within a patient's narrative. Journal of Psychosocial Nursing and Mental Health Services 40: 42–50.

Barker P, Campbell P and Davidson B (1999) From the Ashes of Experience: reflections on recovery, madness and growth. London: Whurr.

Barker P and Kerr B (2000) The Process of Psychotherapy: the journey of discovery. Oxford: Butterworth-Heinemann.

Brown M (1998) The Spiritual Tourist: a personal odyssey through the outer reaches of belief. London: Bloomsbury.

Chödrön P (1994) Start Where You Are: a guide to compassionate living. London: Shambhala.

Clarke I (2002) Editorial: telling the new story. Journal of Critical Psychology, Counselling and Psychotherapy 2(4): 201–202.

Clay S (1999) Madness and reality. In: Barker P, Campbell P and Davidson B (eds) From the Ashes of Experience: reflections on recovery, madness and growth. London: Whurr.

Crick F (1995) The Astonishing Hypothesis. New York: Simon and Schuster.

Culliford L (2002) Spiritual care and psychiatric treatment: an introduction. Advances in Psychiatric Treatment 8: 249–261.

Deegan P (1996) Recovery as a journey of the heart. Psychiatric Rehabilitation Journal 19: 91–97.

Ferguson W (2002) Happiness™. Edinburgh: Canongate Books.

Frankl VE (2000) Man's Search for Ultimate Meaning. Cambridge, MA: Perseus Publishing.

Goddard D (1956) A Buddhist Bible. London: George G Harrap.

Jung CG (1961) Memories, Dreams and Reflections. New York: Vintage.

Karasu TB (1999) Spiritual psychotherapy. American Journal of Psychotherapy 53: 143–161.

Karasu TB (2001) The Psychotherapist as Healer. New York: Jason Aronson.

Karasu TB (2003) The Art of Serenity. New York: Simon and Schuster.

King M (2001) Wrestling with the Angel: a life of Janet Frame. London: Picador/ Macmillan.

Leibrich J (1999) A Gift of Stories: discovering how to deal with mental illness. Dunedin: University of Otago Press/Mental Health Commission.

Leibrich J (2001) Making Space – Spirituality and Mental Health. The Mary Hemingway Rees Memorial Lecture, World Assembly for Mental Health, Vancouver, July.

LeShan L (1999) Cancer as a Turning Point. New York: Plume.

Lewis CS (1961) A Grief Observed. London: Fontana.

Montgomery W (1910) Selections from the Confessions of St Augustine. Cambridge: Cambridge University Press.

Newnes C, Holmes G and Dunn C (2000) This is Madness: a critical look at psychiatry and the future of mental health services. Ross-on-Wye: PCCS Books.

O'Brien JA (1964) Eternal Answers for an Anxious Age. London: WH Allen.

O'Donohue J (1997) Anam Cara: spiritual wisdom from the Celtic world. London: Bantam Books.

Pepper J (1992) How to be Happy. Bath: Gateway Books.

Rose D (2000) A year of care. OpenMind 106(Nov/Dec): 19–20.

Royal College of Psychiatrists (2000) Good Psychiatric Practice. London: Royal College of Psychiatrists.

Storm R (1991) In Search of Heaven on Earth. London: Bloomsbury.

Szasz TS (1996) The Meaning of Mind: language, morality and neuroscience. London: Praeger.

Underhill E (1937) The Spiritual Life. New York: Harper and Brothers.

US Department of Health and Human Services (1999) Mental Health: a report of the Surgeon General – Executive Summary. Rockville, MD: US Department of Health and Human Services, Substance Abuse and Mental Health Services Administration, Center for Mental Health Services, National Institutes of Health, National Institute of Mental Health.

Wallace BA (1989) Choosing Reality: a contemplative view of physics and the mind. Boston, MA: New Science Library Shambhala.

Watts A (1977) The Essential Alan Watts. Berkeley, CA: Celestial Arts.

Whiteside P (2001) Happiness: the 30-day guide. London: Rider Books.

Part Two
Meanings

Nothing is created from a single, original source. I have directly experienced this truth, and you can also. My goal is not to explain the universe, but to help guide others to have a direct experience of reality. Words cannot describe reality. Only direct experience enables us to see the true face of reality.

Thich Nhat Hanh

I do not know whether I was then a man dreaming I was a butterfly, or whether I am now a butterfly dreaming I am a man.

Chuang Tzu

If we can really understand the problem, the answer will come out of it, because the answer is not separate from the problem.

Krishnamurti

CHAPTER 2

Chocolate Cakes

DAVID BRANDON

David Brandon was born in Sunderland and began to run away from home at the age of 13, sleeping rough in Tyneside and London, all the time honing his appreciation of the lifestyle, meaning and value of the outsider. From this rocky soil sprung his lifelong ambition for social work. He also became a counsellor and tireless advocate for compassion in human services. In adult life he became a survivor of psychiatric break-down and psychiatric services, becoming an international authority on services for the homeless and other dispossessed people – from his fellow travellers, the 'mentally ill', to people with learning disabilities. He was ordained as a Buddhist monk in 1982 and ten years later became Professor of Community Care at Anglia Polytechnic University, England, where he inspired countless students to risk thinking in his iconoclastic ways. He died in 2002.

Life is in the baking

One of the most popular pastries we baked was a dense chocolate torte ... it turned out to be delicious and special. Around that time, we hired a professional baker to help us increase our efficiency – and he made a few changes in the way we prepared our Godiva chocolate torte. Almost imme-diately, we got a call from the people at Godiva, and they said, 'What's happened?' In fact it was good. But it was good the way any other choco-late torte was good. It was no longer special ... Experts can be useful ... but ... we had to learn to keep our uniqueness and style ...

Glassman and Fields (1996: 68)

Definitions

Spirituality is an immensely difficult term to define, interwoven with so many other mysterious words like Tao, religion and mysticism. Many see it as indefinable. 'The Tao that can be trodden is not the enduring and unchanging Tao. The name that can be named is not the enduring and unchanging name' (Lao Tzu, 1994: 1). Spirituality could be said to be about finding our basic humanity – the same essence we share with every person. And discovering that, we are finding still more. Words fall short of spiritual experience 'like stones thrown at the stars' (O'Connor and Dermott, 1996: 34). Other more recent authors are bolder but not necessarily any wiser. 'Spirituality is at the ground of our being and seeks to transcend the self and discover belonging and relatedness to the infinite'(Joseph, 1987: 15).

Sacco looks at the seamlessness of spirituality in African life: 'African religion is so integrated as a way of life that African languages have no word for religion as such ... the terms spirituality, religion and theology are used to refer to the same experience' (Sacco, 1996: 46). Sermabeikian offers a more Western view: 'The spiritual perspective requires that we look at the meaning of life, that we look beyond the fear and limitations of the immediate problem with the goal of discovering something inspirational and meaningful rather than focusing on the past and on pathology' (Sermabeikian, 1994).

In one study, a huge majority of social workers (95%) felt that spirituality and religion had distinctly different meanings. Most saw religion as being a group process, associated with formal institutional practices, and spirituality linked with an individual's search for meaning or a 'connection with something greater than one's self' (Derezotes and Evans, 1995: 46).

Some writers see them as virtual opposites. 'The spirituality that emerges spontaneously at a certain stage of experiential self-exploration should not be confused with the mainstream religions and their beliefs, doctrines, dogmas and rituals. Many of them have lost entirely the connection with their original sources, which is a visionary experience of transpersonal realities ... It is possible to have a religion with very little spirituality' (Grof, 1988: 269).

Spirituality moves in the opposite direction from social work, which has increasingly stressed the unique nature of individuality. It is not about separateness but explores the wider connections, uncovering our profoundly common nature. It includes a drive to heal, to bring together the million fragments within us. '... we create a persistent alienation from ourselves, from others, and from the world by fracturing our present experience into different parts, separated by boundaries. We artificially split our awareness into compartments such as subject vs object, life vs death, inside vs outside, reason vs instinct – a divorce settlement that sets experience cutting into experience and life fighting with life' (Wilber, 1979: Preface). Bringing these warring segments together is the spiritual journey.

A lack of clarity about definition is intrinsically charming but very difficult. What exactly are we studying? What is included and excluded? A fuzzy subject can easily be sprayed on almost anything and attracts charlatans in large numbers.

Relevance

Many authors comment on the neglect of and even an antagonism towards the term 'spirituality' (Sermabeikian, 1994; Brandon, 1996; Canda, 1988; Joseph, 1988). 'Mental health practitioners have an almost negative reaction to the introduction of the word "spirituality" into clinical discussions' (Cornett, 1992). In practice, the situation can be even worse than that. These age-old elements have become largely pathologized. 'The only framework available for a direct experience of alternative realities of a spiritual nature has been, until recently, that of mental disease' (Grof, 1985: 367).

Although explored in many social work 'values modules', religion and spirituality don't form a part of the record of everyday practice and are rarely discussed in practice seminars. They tend to be left to one side in work with clients. Lloyd argues fervently against 'an automatic "sectioning off" of spiritual pain from everything else by social workers' and notes, reasonably, that nursing literature has paid greatest attention to a spiritual dimension' (Lloyd, 1997). Barker seems to cast some doubt on that: 'What may be controversial is my belief that psychiatric nursing is a spiritual activity; that nurses participate in the psychic healing of the person with mental illness' (Barker, 1996.)

Despite its relative neglect in textbooks, spirituality remains influential in professional practice. Ninety-one per cent of social work students in a South African survey saw it providing 'the opportunity to be part of the collective; guidance; clarity; a perspective on life; direction; sustenance; a growing to wholeness ... and a reminder of the ever-presence of God' (Sacco, 1996: 52).

In the West, at least in the fuzzy New Age circles, spirituality has become fashionable. It is perceived as something precious and highly desirable, like fine chocolate powder spread over a stodgy pudding to give a special flavour. Take this passage from a popular counselling text:

> It is clear to me now that the decision to trust the feeling of interrelatedness was the first step towards a willingness on my part to acknowledge my

spiritual experience of reality and to capitalise on the many hours spent in prayer and worship. It was as if previously I had refused to draw on this whole area of awareness in the conduct of my therapeutic work. In my zeal not to proselytise it was as if I had deliberately deprived myself of some of the most precious resources in the task of relating to my clients. Once I had opened myself to myself, however, I was capable of experiencing the communion of souls, or the membership of one of another, which is the fundamental given of the spiritual life.

Mearns and Thorne (1988)

Note carefully the language used – 'my spiritual experience' is to be 'capitalised' on. Phrases like 'my clients', 'opened myself to myself', 'to trust the feeling of interrelatedness' sound not like the music of spirituality but of inflating egos, the use of a crude tool applied to the client. Nothing in the language of spirituality prepares the student for a box of hammers and spanners.

Whatever its meaning, many writers claim a revival of interest in the profession. 'Many people are searching for spiritual meaning and an ontological significance in their lives ... The religious movement is beginning to make its appearance felt in professional social work thinking and education for practice ...' (Siporin, 1985). It is unclear yet whether this is a fervent wish or a practical reality. I note no great surge of genuine interest but rather a simple changing of fashions; wooden beads rather than spiritual quest.

Spirituality as psychotherapy?

Eigen, a psychoanalyst, comments: 'I've spoken at a number of conferences on spirituality and psychotherapy the last several years, and at each one a Buddhist has ... said that practising Buddhist meditation can shorten psychotherapy by years ... I find it fruitless to pit religion and psychotherapy against each other. I find it especially cruel for either religion or psychotherapy to advertise itself as an agent for that which it can't deliver' (Eigen, 1998: 163). How very right he is. This is a false battle we really don't need.

Meditation is frequently offered as a psychotherapeutic technique, everything from psychoanalytic to behaviourist, mostly a de luxe brand:

If people can be taught to recognize their thoughts, feelings and anxieties as they arise, if they can develop greater tolerance of frustration and stress, if they can be shown how to relax more easily, if they can be given skills to control their sensations, then these will contribute towards the prevention of at least some of the common psychological disorders. The

behavioural and cognitive techniques that Buddhism offers, particularly but
not exclusively in meditation, seem eminently suitable for such a role.

De Silva (1984)

However, the spiritual road is not a psychotherapeutic motorway. It has
very little to do with personal growth or achievement and has other purposes and processes. Such a road is widely and sometimes even wilfully
misunderstood and its means subverted. Aguilar comments: '... social
workers have secularised the search for the sacred by recodifying the concept as personal transformation, self-fulfilment, or self-esteem' (Aguilar,
1997). We have taken these ancient and wise traditions and beaten and
twisted them into a personal growth framework in to which they fit
uneasily.

This predominant framework insists that everybody should and can be
fixed. It is the unceasing search for new syndromes, the pathologization
of the whole universe. 'In principle, there is an assumption that all human
problems can be converted into technical problems, and if the techniques
to solve certain problems do not yet exist, then they will have to be
invented. The world becomes ever more "makeable"' (Berger, 1977: 36).
We are surrounded by ever-increasing numbers of psychological plumbers
and mechanics.

Our world is permeated with mechanistic metaphors. For example,
those in poverty, the homeless and disabled – the socially excluded – are
seen as the other. 'Our attitudes towards society's most deprived out-
siders are mechanistic attitudes, if we perceive them as wholly other, as
objectives of our pity and fear, as a problem to be overcome or a threat to
be defended against, these attitudes may evoke the behaviour that we
most fear, the rage and violence that do indeed threaten us, our property
and our daily activities' (Zohar and Marshal, 1994). They become deval-
ued people.

The spiritual way points in quite another direction, stressing respect
and valuing for all. None of us are experts in daily living. Zen particularly
demands the shedding of opinions and expertise rather than in more
intellectual accumulation. When much younger I knew a great deal, now
closer to retirement, I'm constantly amazed by how little I know.

Sowaki Roshi said: 'To gain is illusion, to lose is enlightenment'
(Brandon, 1982a). This calls for the radically different posture of *Begin-
ner's Mind*. 'How might an empty mind be used in psychiatric nursing
practice? I can only speak from my own experience. For some time I have
been part of a family team offering to meet with people *characterized* as
having severe and enduring mental health problems who are also usually
veterans of psychiatric services. Rather than "therapying", we try to offer
speculative comments to the people, which they may, or may not, find

interesting. Early in my new experience, I found myself striving to divest myself of the belief that the theories that had been part of my profession-al socialization were more real, helpful, truthful than other, more vicariously adopted ideas. By doing so, I found that I could be more cre-ative, playful, and interesting for the people who were listening' (Stevenson, 1996). Divesting oneself of the heavy pressure to be a top expert, it is easy to find illuminated energy.

Rather more prosaically, Zen Master Glassman describes a Buddhist retreat spent homeless on New York streets: 'None of us really wound up suffering. We were not experiencing homelessness. We all knew we were going back home after four days. But we were experiencing living in an environment that forced us to forget about all other aspects of life and made us deal directly with eating, sleeping and surviving. One night we slept in boxes we found on the street. It was cold, the pavement was hard, the streetlights were shining, and there was noise all night. The street stripped us bare' (Glassman and Fields, 1996: 167). I had experience of living rough in London as a teenager running away from a violent home. The rain and cold stripped me of any ideas and even hopes.

Self-improvement, personal growth, individual or personal success have little connection with spirituality. They consist of achieving and get-ting – not in simply being. The spiritual pathway presents no academic argument, crushing opponents with skills and wit. It smells the plums, hears the rain, and sometimes loves others and sometimes not.

> Alone in mountain fastness,
> Dozing by the window.
> No mere talk uncovers Truth:
> The fragrance of those garden plums.
>
> Bankei quoted in Brandon (1990: 5)

It means just living in this world as best we can. Soon after the death of Rabbi Moshe, Rabbi Mendel of Kotzk asked one of his disciples: 'What was most important to your teacher?' The disciple thought and replied: 'Whatever he happened to be doing at the moment' (Buber, 1948: 173). Some of us are lions and others dandelions. Which is better? A silly question. Is it for gos-samering in summer breezes or hunting a herd of wildebeest?

Wilkes comes closest to solving the improved chocolate cake paradox. 'The aim of life is not the achievement of some purpose thought up by others, but the achievement of individuality. If life is for the living, the focus should not be on correction but on appreciation; life must be appreciated even when there is nothing to correct' (Wilkes, 1983: 18). Just two caveats – there is nothing to be achieved in that sense, only some-thing to realized; and there is, on one level, no real individuality either, biologically or psychologically.

Temptations

There is a great temptation to see spirituality as something superbly special, as some sort of superior power. It is often written about as if containing the most superior qualities, ingredients surpassing all others, possessed only by a chosen few people, close to perfection. '... one of the ways in which "spirit" has been interpreted is to separate it altogether from organised religion and a set of beliefs and link it to a "special way of being". Spirit and spiritual states are seen as something beyond the mundane and everyday' (Petrioni, 1993). Such a quest for perfection is destructive whether in chocolate cakes or gurus.

This Disney magnet – the temptation to beautify – to concentrate exclusively on the light rather than the darkness, is extremely powerful and injurious. 'As a finite self, then, a human struggles to find goodness, truth, beauty and life at the exclusion of evil, falsity, ugliness and death. But such one-sided fulfillment is impossible. Given the inseparability of the poles, one cannot arrive at a pure or absolute form of one pole at the exclusion of the other. Although someone might find temporary, relative satisfaction, the negation of that satisfaction soon arises. Expressed with the metaphor of waves, insofar as people exist as waves on the agitated surface of an expanse of water, they are eternally unsettled, for waves continue to arise and fall in endless opposition' (Ives, 1992: 74).

Inevitably it is discovered that these so-called 'perfect individuals chew tobacco, drink too much, are fond of sex with beautiful men and women'. My *Guardian* newspaper informs me this week, rather late, that Kahlil Gibran, author of the best-selling book *The Prophet* was a womanizer and an alcoholic:

NEW AGE GURU WAS AGE OLD HYPOCRITE

Millar (1998)

So bloody what? Why do spiritual teachers have to be perfect? The worship of false idols – and all idols are false – is both dangerous and destructive. The Zen Masters and Tibetan lamas I've known have been ordinary men and women shrouded in projected mystery, capable of great heights and extraordinary stupidities. Nothing special. My first Zen teacher asked through a cloud of cigarette smoke: 'David you would prefer it if I didn't smoke?' I nodded affirmatively. She responded just as quickly: 'Tough luck.' It was a profound teaching. She was realizing the truth of George Orwell's remark of Gandhi: 'No doubt alcohol, tobacco and so forth are things that a saint must avoid, but sainthood is also a thing that human beings must avoid' (Lomas, 1987:12).

It is so easy to get fluffy about spirituality. The paradoxes can get filled with mystical nonsense. Much of what passes for contemporary spirituality is linked with the New Age movement, characterized by promiscuity – borrowing and stealing from hundreds of different disciplines. This can result in an unhealthy sprint from reason, taking refuge in a sloppy fudge of sentimentality and hugging; the widespread public grieving over Princess Diana is such an excellent example. Our yearnings for spirituality can invent yet another commodity, an improved product with fresh ingredients.

This problem is not at all new. Richard Hooker, the sixteenth-century preacher, commented: 'Hence an error groweth, when men in heaviness of spirit suppose they lack faith, because they find not the sugared joy and delight which indeed doth accompany faith, but so as a separable accident, as a thing that may be removed from it; yea there is a cause why it should be removed. The light would never be acceptable, were it not for that usual intercourse of darkness. Too much honey doth turn to gall; and too much joy even spiritually would make us wantons. Happier a great deal is that man's case, whose soul by inward desolation is humbled, than he whose heart is through abundance of spiritual delight lifted up and exalted above measure' (Keble, 1845).

Spiritual gifts can and are easily used for essentially egotistical purposes. We can subvert even the noblest of intentions. Sawaki Roshi comments brusquely: 'to do good can be bad. There are people who do good deeds to adorn themselves ... Everything turns on whether one believes in religion in order to improve oneself or whether one lets go of the mind that wants to gain something. The former is a heretic who exploits God and the Buddha, and the latter is a truly religious person' (Uchiyama, 1990).

To Buddhists, spirituality is a journey towards realizing the absence of barriers: 'that one is all things: mountains, rivers, grasses, trees, sun, moon, stars, universe, are all oneself ... Realizing this naturally results in what we commonly refer to in Zen Buddhism as "true compassion". Other people and things are no longer seen as apart from oneself, but, on the contrary, as one's own body' (Merzel, 1991). This is the essential harmony of ordinary, everyday living rather than some devotion to self-cherishing.

Trungpa, the late Tibetan lama, rightly warned against the immense dangers of self-improvement. 'It means that whatever we do with our practice, if that practice is connected with our personal achievement, which is called "spiritual materialism", or the individual glory that we are in the right and others are wrong, and we would like to conquer their wrongness or evil because we are on the side of God and so forth – that kind of bullshit or cow dung is regarded as eating poisonous food. Such food may be presented to us beautifully and nicely, but when we begin to eat it, it stinks' (Trungpa, 1993: 178). We have to be even more scrupulous about so-called good intentions than we are about so-called bad ones. Most of us have damaged someone we loved, through idiot compassion.

The late Ruth Picardie wrote concretely: 'Worse than the God botherers, though, are the road accident rubber-neckers, who seem to find terminal illness exciting, the secular Samaritans looking for glory. Hey, I met you once three years ago but can we do lunch so I can feel really good about myself when I read your obituary? *Yeah.* I know we lost touch four years ago, but can I be your best friend again so everyone will feel sorry for me at the funeral?' (Picardie, 1998: 73). God save me from God botherers and rubber-neckers who seem to haunt the hospitals.

We can easily misuse and abuse the power and energy coming from genuine attempts to heal. 'In general, the power drive is given freest rein when it can appear under the cloak of objective and moral rectitude. People are the most cruel when they can use cruelty to enforce the "good" (Guggenbuhl-Craig, 1971: 10). Insensitivity is rather more common than cruelty. Picardie again on social workers: 'I had begun to think of them as self-sacrificing super-heroes second only to comprehensive teachers. That was until last week, when I was allocated one of my own. Alerted by the local social services that my "care needs" were to be assessed by a member of the disability team, I became, well, perhaps not incandescent, but certainly breathless and headachey with rage. How *dare* they. How dare some *stranger* come barging into my house, snooping around and passing judgement – after only the most superficial of acquaintances – on whether I was sick enough to merit a subsidised cleaner' (Picardie, 1998: 42).

Simpler still is the temptation to emphasize one's own consummate competence at the considerable expense of the clients. Thus according to the Rabbi of GER, 'the single most important issue in the rabbi–client relationship is how the rabbi deals with the potential for arrogance when people come to him for answers and he resists the temptation to "rattle them off", so as to speak, to the client' (Polsky and Wozner, 1989: 78).

Kavan

It's lunchtime, though as I'm on this Draconian diet to shift a sagging stomach, my plate is empty. I'm making a midday meal at very short notice for a large friend who has physical disabilities. One of his personal assistants has dropped out at short notice for sketchy reasons. I am struggling to heat a prepared dish of minced beef and pasta, which, as I am a vegetarian, is a considerable sacrifice of principle.

I am fuming inside. A well-known professor of community care with more than 170 published works to his credit is making lunch for a man with a disability while a dozen research projects await. But as a recompense I gain large numbers of Brownie points and gold stars. I am far away from the imagined ivory towers inhabited by academics. I am working at the real coalface in the real world where it's all happening, while other social work tutors, God help them, bend arthritically over their computers and move mountains of paper from one side of their desks to the other in between attending the interminable meetings.

Kavan keeps asking me: 'Who was supposed to do my lunch? Who's dropped out? I am unhappy about this.' He's unhappy! What about me? Dragged away at five minutes' notice from my office and struggling with a dumb microwave oven. I take his lunch to the tray on the wheelchair for the third time. 'It's still cold,' he grimaces. Whatever my limited skills as a social work teacher, I'm useless as a cook. These banal practicalities are the test, not the ability to write books or do research.

For the seventh time: 'Who should be doing my lunch?' I really don't know and really don't care one bit. Boringly he tells me once more that he's unhappy. I know he's unhappy. I struggle again with the microwave having just failed to find any potatoes. Kavan has a marvellously subtle way of requesting something and when you can't comply, responding with an implication of incompetence, honed over many years in residential care. The potatoes must be there, it's just that I'm too stupid to see them.

I'm now chock-full of rage. I'm so angry with him because he asks the same question over and over again to which I don't know the answer. I know it's memory loss due to the head injury. I'm beginning to feel that I should know. My anger rattles around the cutlery drawer. Now I can't find anything, even the napkins. Kavan asks very pointedly how I became a professor. He seems bemused rather than fascinated. It obviously didn't include microwave oven or potato tests, as I take his meal out once more and simultaneously explain about the obligatory oral exam – for the professorship, not the cooking.

He's deeply angry too – stuck in that bloody wheelchair while the real world goes by outside. From the promise of a young soldier playing prop forward for Cheshire rugby union team to life in a wheelchair, seldom going out. Planned routines, an important aspect of his everyday life, are just broken and disregarded by thoughtless others. Waiting all day for a social worker who never comes because she's too busy. Sacred staffing rotas are ignored and unexpected professors dumped on you and even the microwave mounts dumb resistance.

I know a thousand clever tricks from psychotherapy training and social work to process and juggle this anger. I can envision pink flamingos flying over the African plains; hear light waltz music to relax tense tissues;

do yoga asanas on my neck; punish myself with an ideological birch for falling short of the 150 social work lunch preparation competencies – from empathy to communication skills.

I choose none of the above. The immense anger surges up my body almost to choking. After a brief period of this surge, I can feel Kavan's frustration every time he speaks both in the overtones and undertones. Some comes from the immense disappointment about life in a wheelchair, having to depend on frequently unreliable people making your lunch, while mine comes from a childhood of poverty and my Dad daily beating me up.

'Would you like some peas?' I ask. I can find a packet of peas but no potatoes. 'Yes,' he responds, and like a demented parrot, 'but who was supposed to do my lunch? Where are they? I'm unhappy.' For the umpteenth time I respond that I don't know. I wish I did know. It's an extremely large part of the human condition to be unhappy. It arises out of the great disappointment that life isn't the way it ought to be. The person who is supposed to prepare the lunch didn't show – didn't care enough; didn't follow the script. Kavan and I share that disappointment in spades. Who are we and who is unhappy?

When I've finished all these ideological ramblings, simply a major distraction, there's still the lunch to get. The damned microwave is infuriating. None of the buttons seems to work. Why do machines always make me feel so stupid? He's hungry and so am I. Spin-dryer mind whirls round and round again. Anger; healthy eating or rather not eating; accumulating lots of Brownie points; unhappiness; should be somewhere else; deep disappointment in not being a good enough person; should feel warm compassion for Kavan but don't at present; return reluctantly to the discipline of mindful practice, come back into the kitchen and attend to the lunch. This final time the minced beef and veg meets the Kavan test but only just. 'Can I have some more coffee?' I make the coffee and then there's all the washing up to do.

> The Great Way is not difficult
> for those who don't pick or choose.
> When love and hate are both absent
> everything becomes clear and undistinguished.
> Make the smallest distinction, however
> and heaven and earth are set infinitely apart.
> If you wish to see the truth
> then hold no opinions for or against anything.
>
> Sengstan 'Hsin Hsin Ming' in Brandon (1982b)

I wonder what that old sixth-century Zen monk Sengstan, in far off China, meant by all that?

Conclusion

It is so easy to get self-righteous and stupid. Humility is a rare human quality. 'I'm more holistic than thou' is best avoided. We do need to take things
apart, to ask shrewder questions, but also to avoid the pitfalls of self-cherishing. The Zen pathway points to an essential unity, a desire for holism.
But definitely not as some unattainable Holy Grail; rather as an ever-pres-
ent reality, which we don't usually recognize. The healing takes place from
where we are, not from where we might like to be. We need to turn away
from trying to become gods and goddesses and be what we already are.

At the basis of all healing, for which we are simply a vehicle, is increasing self-awareness and compassion towards others. Nothing very special.
This asks that we are increasingly gentle with ourselves and with others;
that we recognize in our hearts our connectedness; that we surrender our
different images of perfection as a deluded measure of the world and see
it with honesty and love. As Sawaki Roshi commented: 'Everybody is in his
own dream. The discrepancies that exist between the dreams are the
problem' (Uchiyama, 1990: 75). Kavan and I have different scripts but
almost certainly from the same play. In our heads, things are supposed to
run smoothly and coherently, but very seldom do. We need to experience
and look at the frustrations, which emerge from the large gap between
'supposed to' and actual life, and how and why we are both bewildered
and disappointed by life's constant 'imperfections'.

Homer's Odysseus turns away from perfection. The goddess Calypso,
who saved his life and tended him lovingly, entreats him not to join his
wife, Penelope, in Ithaca. My lady goddess, do not be angry at what I am
about to say. I too know well enough that my wise Penelope's looks and
stature are insignificant compared with yours. For she is mortal, while you
have immortality and unfading youth. Nevertheless I long to reach my
home and see the day of my return. It is my never-failing wish. And what
if one of the gods does wreck me on the wine-dark sea? I have a heart that
is inured to suffering and I shall steel it to endure that too. For in my day
I have had many bitter and painful experiences in war and on the stormy
seas. So let this disaster come. It only makes one more.

He rejects the likelihood of enduring love and immortality; chooses his
wife, Penelope, rather than Calypso; chooses his human heritage – the
ordinary life of a Greek hero – with the triumphs and disasters, the sickness, dying and eventual death. Would he make that choice again today?
In our age of plastic surgery, the dawn of cloning and the invention of a
hundred thousand psychological tricks and techniques, I believe he
would refuse the quest for perfection in favour of ordinary living. Those
of us travelling the same road must firmly resist the temptation to bake
the perfect chocolate cake on Ithaca or anywhere else. Our spiritual path-

way is about uncovering more of who we are, rather than in striving for what or who we might be.

References

Aguilar M (1997) Re-engineering social work's approach to holistic healing. Health and Social Work 22(2): 83.

Barker P (1996) The logic of experience: developing appropriate care through effective collaboration. Australian and New Zealand Journal of Mental Health Nursing 5: 3–12.

Berger PL (1977) Pyramids of Sacrifice. New York: Basic Books.

Brandon D (1982a) Simply Meditate. Preston, England: Tao.

Brandon D (1982b) Beginning Zen. Preston, England: Tao.

Brandon D (1990) Zen in the Art of Helping. London: Penguin.

Brandon D (1996) Spirituality in social work practice teaching. Issues in Social Work Education 16(2): 71–79.

Buber M (1948) Tales of the Hassidim – the later Masters vol II. New York: Schocken Books.

Canda ER (1988) Conceptualizing spirituality for social work: insights from diverse perspectives. Social Thought 13: 30–46.

Cornett C (1992) Toward a more comprehensive personology; integrating a spiritual perspective into social work practice. Social Work 37(2): 101.

De Silva P (1984) Buddhism and behaviour modification. Behaviour Research and Therapy 6: 661–678.

Derezotes DS and Evans KR (1995) Spirituality and religiosity in practice: in-depth interviews of social work practitioners. Social Thought 18(1): 39–54.

Eigen M (1998) The Psychoanalytic Mystic. New York: Free Association Books.

Glassman B and Fields R (1996) Instructions to the Cook – a Zen Master's lessons in living a life that matters. New York: Bell Tower.

Grof S (1985) Beyond the Brain. New York: State University of New York.

Grof S (1988) The Adventure of Self-Discovery. New York: State University of New York.

Guggenbuhl-Craig A (1971) Power in the Helping Professions. London: Spring Publications.

Ives C (1992) Zen Awakening and Society. London: Macmillan.

Joseph MV (1987) The religious and spiritual aspects of clinical practice: a neglected dimension of social work. Social Thought 3: 12–23.

Joseph MV (1988) Religion and social work practice. Social Casework, September: 443–452.

Keble J (ed.) (1845) The Works of that Learned and Judicious Divine, Mr Richard Hooker, 3rd edn, vol. III. Oxford: Oxford University Press, pp. 474–475.

Lloyd M (1997) Dying and bereavement. Spirituality and social work in a market economy of welfare. British Journal of Social Work 27(2): 175–190.

Lomas P (1987) Quotes from George Orwell: 'Reflections on Gandhi'. In: The Limits of Interpretation. London: Penguin.

Mearns D and Thorne B (1988) Person-Centred Counselling in Action. London: Sage.

Merzel DG (1991) The Eye Never Sleeps: striking to the heart of Zen. Boston, MA: Shambala.

Millar S (1998) New Age Guru was age old hypocrite. The Guardian 22 June: 5.

O'Connor J and Dermott TI (1996) Principles of NLP. London: Thorsons.

Petrioni P (1993) The return of the spirit. In: Beattie A (ed.) Health and Well Being – a reader. Basingstoke: Macmillan and Open University.

Picardie R (1998) Before I Say Goodbye. London: Penguin.

Polsky HW and Wozner Y (1989) Everyday Miracles – the healing wisdom of Hassidic stories. Northvale, NJ: Aronson.

Sacco T (1996) Spirituality and social work students in South Africa. Journal of Social Development in Africa 11(2): 43–56.

Sermabeikian P (1994) Our clients, ourselves: the spiritual perspective and social work practice. Social Work 39(2): 145–240.

Siporin M (1985) Current social work perspectives on clinical practice. Clinical Social Work Journal 13(3): 198–217.

Stevenson C (1996) The Tao, social constructionism and psychiatric nursing practice and research. Journal of Psychiatric and Mental Health Nursing 3(4): 41–49.

Trungpa C (1993) Training the Mind. Boston, MA: Shambala.

Lao Tzu (1994) Tao Te Ching (Streep P ed.). Boston, MA: Bullfinch Press.

Uchiyama K (1990) The Zen Teaching of 'Homeless' Kodo. Tokyo: Schumucho, pp. 67–68.

Wilber K (1979) No Boundary – Eastern and Western approaches to personal growth. New York: Center Publications.

Wilkes R (1983) Social Work with Undervalued Groups. London: Tavistock.

Zohar D and Marshall I (1994) The Quantum Society. London: Flamingo.

CHAPTER 3

Perceptions of Reality

ANNE DRYSDALE

Anne Drysdale writes:

> Significant events in my life during 1984 granted me an affinity with others who had experienced or believed in a spiritual reality. I subsequently found myself, late in life, moving into formal education, studying subjects relating to religion and spirituality – concluding with an MA dissertation on 'Perceptions of Spiritual and Psychotic Experience'. I was delighted, therefore, to accept an invitation to contribute to this book and pray that the words will touch at least someone, somewhere.

Introduction

Because of the personal nature and wide variety of sensations and reactions produced by spiritual experience, the concept of spirituality can only be authentically defined according to the individual's own spiritual awareness; but in simplistic terms, what basically sets spiritual experience apart from other experiences is its unrelatedness to materialism.

The poet John Donne visualizes spirituality as the link between humanity and divinity, rejecting the idea that any human being lives in isolation. Donne's belief that 'No man is an island, entire of itself', offers a spiritual lifeline to those who feel alone and possibly forsaken. Could it be, however, that despite making this potentially redemptive, life-enhancing connection with a non-physical reality, some experiencers are subsequently drawn into the psychiatric system, misunderstood and eventually diagnosed psychotic, as a result of an inability to cope with either their reactions to the experience(s) or their frustration at incomprehension and consequent negative responses from hearers, or a combination of both?

Summary

Due to our individual, enclosed mindsets – causing the perceived isolation to which Donne refers – each one of us develops a totally personal
viewpoint from which a unique concept of life on earth is ultimately
formed; although even personal perceptions are subject to fluctuation
and division as the child, and then adult, becomes affected by a wealth of
experiences during the journey through life. Consequently, the accumu-
lated perceptions offered for consideration in this chapter are inevitably
drawn from an individual life history, subject to a particular personality
and under the influence of all the various impressions made on the mind,
heart and soul of the writer.

These perceptions will be presented in the form of an imaginary spiritual journey, with the character of Grace adopted as a medium to explore
the causes and effects of personal reactions to life experiences, focusing
on those of a spiritual nature. It will be argued that Grace's particular personality traits and deviation from an ingrained moral code were the
primary factors in her difficulties with personal relationships and subsequent emotional problems, leading eventually to a mental crisis. The
important role of hearers in their response to reported other world experiences will also be considered.

Spiritual 'seeds'

We all react to life on earth according to our own unique thought patterns, created by the information fed to us via the experiences occurring
throughout our lives. For some reason, certain experiences or incidents
make a deep and lasting impression, and though the thought placed in
the mind may lie dormant – perhaps for a lifetime – something deep within the person has been touched, waiting to be recalled when the time is
right. Such experiences can occur early in life, young children being generally more open and receptive to experiences of another world – a
fantasy world beyond the limits of the one in which they normally live.

An attempt to describe Grace's early spiritual experience would not
explain the extraordinariness of it. A child making her way to primary
school, eyes drawn towards the sky as the clouds parted, allowing a bright
light to envelop her in its rays, would be regarded as simply a blink of sunshine; but Grace's reaction to the experience defies such a simplistic
explanation. She immediately felt a sensation of tremendous joy – a sense
of joy unlike anything previously experienced; an experience she kept
enclosed within her mind and one she could still vividly recall late in her
life. The comment of a contributor to Alister Hardy's research on spiritual

experiences suggests that what happened to Grace was the foundation for future similar events: 'It is only today, gathering up the threads as it were, that I realise that this childhood experience set the pattern for subsequent ones' (Hardy, 1997: 104).

The mind of a young child is fertile ground for new ideas which stir the imagination. Children love stories and never tire of hearing their favourites repeated. The film version of *Pinocchio*, with his guiding 'conscience' in the form of Jiminy Cricket, a popular film when Grace was a child, had a significant effect on her. As the film story implies, the human conscience is the seat of morality. Grace was reminded of Jiminy Cricket much later in her life when the writings of a Scottish theologian were brought to her attention. Thomas Erskine believed that 'All spiritual truth is addressed to the conscience' (Hanna, 1878: 401).

Erskine conceives of two powers within every human being, symbolized as flesh and spirit, which are seeds sown within, but separate from each individual. His theory is that the onus is on every human being to make a personal choice between the two powers – the power of evil (things of self), or the power of good (the Spirit). William James presents a similar, though less theological, view that some people '... refuse to believe, their personal energy never gets to its religious centre, and the latter remains inactive in perpetuity' (James, 1982: 204). Both theories place the onus or choice on the individual: a reference to human free will.

The father figure in the story of Pinocchio personifies the loving God of the Christian faith, planting a softer, more spiritual message into the young mind than that of the religious teaching she received. The predominant features of traditional Christian teaching during Grace's childhood were the sinfulness of human nature, with emphasis on 'thou shalt nots', and the written word; the latter certainly being an important point of reference for any religion, but not if used as 'dead letter'. Although sweeping changes are taking place today, the spiritual aspect of Christianity has been sadly neglected – a side effect of the Reformation and dissolution of the monasteries.

With the approach of adulthood, Grace reacted to religious instruction with increasing feelings of guilt at any perceived deviation from the strict moral code. Her 'strings', like those of the puppet, were manipulated by others, drawing her at times into spiritually regressive situations. Nevertheless, for some, the disciplines of traditional Christianity appear to meet their needs. Others, following spiritual experience, become aware of the deviation from its roots and the consequent lack of spirituality in traditional religious teaching, as occurred with Grace.

Children are soon introduced to the attractions of the material world, and Grace was no exception. As she grew into adulthood, the memory of the moral message, given in the form of Jiminy Cricket, faded – though sheltered somewhere in the recesses of her mind was a compelling desire to search for answers; mostly on the question of love. Her search, however, was focused on the material world and, as a result, she gradually moved into an emotional and mental minefield.

Spirituality and intellect

Some research into the background and status of those who report positive spiritual experiences concludes that a high percentage of experiencers are well educated and from good social backgrounds. In his study of spiritual and psychotic experience, Michael Jackson states that the quality of childhood '...influences the tone and content of both pathological and benign adult psychotic and spiritual experiences' (Jackson, 1991: 313). The psychotic sufferers he interviewed had experienced severe emotional problems as children, whereas the group of benign spiritual experients came from more stable backgrounds. Grace's circumstances agree with this conclusion, her early environment and family situation having been 'normal', apart from some conflict between different personalities. She did not, however, move into an intellectual stream, her formal education being very limited; but is this important in relation to spiritual experience?

Connecting spirituality with intellect is challenged by reports from those who lack formal education or have limited intellectual abilities, yet claim to have gained knowledge of the mysteries of the universe. Although William Blake is an exceptional case, as one who spent much of his time 'conversing with angels', his life and work have become subjects of intensive study, despite lack of schooling in early life and, at least, some rejection of reason and intellect as the mediators of his visionary experiences. Jacob Boehme, whose writings greatly influenced Blake, and Joan of Arc, are other visionaries of humble birth and lack of formal education who continue, centuries later, to influence others. Joan claimed to receive instructions from her 'voices', but from what source or 'reality' did Blake and Boehme gain their profound insight to the mysteries of life and knowledge of the universe?

In spite of Blake's reaction to the inspiration for his engraving work as being '... drunk with intellectual vision' (Keynes, 1979: 852), he said of his poems *Milton* and *Jerusalem* that they had been dictated to him – '... the Authors are in Eternity' (Keynes, 1979: 825). Without any effort or study, he claims to have produced epic works, which would normally have been the labour of a lifetime. Such a statement defies reason and does not conform to accepted definitions of sanity; yet the enduring quality of the visionary's writings testifies to their content of truth.

From his research into the spiritual nature of humanity, Alister Hardy concludes that: 'The spirit of man is not the product of intellectuality' (Hardy, 1997: 140). This theory is reinforced by David Hay's reference to the work of Henri Bissonier, '... who writes about the profound spiritual awareness he has observed in people who are mentally retarded' (Hay, 1998: 51). Jean Vanier, the founder of the L'Arche communities where the mentally handicapped live in communion with their assistants, is also one who is aware of positive aspects of mental retardation. In an article about the community, the journalist comments on the spiritual element at its core, which provides a haven of peace, strength and stability from which both care workers and the handicapped draw.

The implication is not, of course, that intellectuals are less likely to experience the spirit world – in fact, it seems most likely that more reports come from the well educated, due to their ability to express themselves. Rather, spirituality cannot be experienced by rational means and so the simple minded and uneducated have equal, or perhaps easier, access to spiritual awareness. Grace's limited formal education, therefore, was irrelevant to the spiritual experiences that occurred in her life; but what caused the emotional problems leading eventually to a mental crisis?

The unstable personality

Individual personality undoubtedly exerts a significant influence on our general attitude to life and reactions to the problems inevitably encountered during our period here on earth. Alister Hardy goes so far as to suggest that personality is the immortal part of each human being: 'I believe we should examine the evidence for the alleged survival of human "personality" after death' (Hardy, 1978: 186). If this theory has any validity, then an important – even primary – reason for our spiritual journey on earth is to mould, reshape, transform or whatever action is required to fit that personality for a particular purpose. It is an understandable view held by some that we should just learn to accept ourselves as we are, warts and all, but if what we are causes unhappiness, mental distress or psychosis, is a change which has the potential to improve our lives, and consequently our relationships with others, not to be desired?

It is difficult for the naturally good-natured, optimistic or extrovert character, who is able to brush off personal setbacks, to understand the complexities that arise in the minds of those of a more introvert personality and nervous disposition, such as Grace. Easily discouraged, but with consoling bright intervals when on a 'high', she was confused by the contrasting effects of uncontrollable emotions while, at the same time, feeling trapped in her situation. Pinocchio's manipulated strings – over which he had no control – and a frustrating desire to be set free depicts, to some extent, Grace's situation. She unconsciously longed for harmony between the sensations of her heart and mind.

Self-consciousness – basically a fear of others – created in Grace feelings of self-doubt and discontent with the persona, or mask, she wore for the world. Although her inner world was unbalanced, Grace's usually calm and confident exterior gave the impression all was well, but the strain of maintaining a 'false' self, aggravated by frustrating, long-standing relationship problems and feelings of guilt, brought intermittent bouts of deep depression. Being extremely sensitive to atmosphere when in company, Grace often negatively 'imagined' what others thought of her and consequently moved deeper into her shell.

For the mentally unstable, whether or not diagnosed psychotic (Grace being in the latter category), emotional life is subject to ever-changing moods, even though the world around remains the same. The phrase 'Windmills of the mind' aptly illustrates extremely sensitive, loosely formed emotions, blown about according to the whims and varying degrees of force and impact from outside influences. In some respects, life would appear to be more exciting and adventurous for the individual with this type of personality. Indeed, during a 'high', when certainty and confidence prevail, anything seems possible to achieve, but 'lows' completely obliterate self-confidence. The insecurity and vulnerability experienced at such times pushes the sufferer inexorably towards the edge of what seems like a bottomless pit – a drop into oblivion.

The terror and panic induced by such a terrifying ordeal can really only be understood by those who have trod this hellish borderland between sanity and madness. The sufferer's acute fear makes him cling on for dear life, like a passenger on a sinking ship. Some remain suspended in this checkmate hell-on-earth situation, afraid to move in any direction; others who set sail on the sea of madness are finally shipwrecked – washed up, shattered into pieces on a foreign shore, as the human spirit is broken and, in some cases, reset.

It is almost impossible to conceive of a more traumatic situation than being faced with this 'threshold'. RD Laing describes the dilemma in existentialist terms, and acknowledges that whether or not the outcome of the experience is insanity depends on reaction to it: 'It will require an act of imagination from those who do not know from their own experience what hell this borderland between being and nonbeing can become. One's posture or stance in relation to the act or process can become decisive from the point of view of madness or sanity' (Laing, 1967: 36).

William James describes the onset of a horrible fear of his own existence, a fear of non-being, induced by the image of an 'entirely idiotic ... absolutely non-human' epileptic patient he had seen in an asylum. The psychologist's fear arose from the thought 'That shape *am I* ... potentially' (James, 1982: 160). He reveals that only by clinging to scriptural texts was he prevented from becoming really insane. Carl Jung claimed to have discovered a wealth of knowledge from psychic experience; but he too encountered the 'threshold' during his seven-year journey into near madness following his break with Freud: 'It was only towards the end of the First World War that I gradually began to emerge from the darkness' (Jung, 1983: 220). William Blake was also subject to treading the sane/mad borderland.

James' negative experience gave him insight into the concept of madness, yet he managed to hold on to his sanity despite the horrifying effects of the experience. However, Blake's visionary experiences were, for him, extremely positive; he was aware that he was different from others in his perception, '... but in his opinion the deficiency was theirs and not his, evidence of their entrapment in a material hell' (Youngquist, 1989: 14). If, as he claimed, Blake's visionary experiences were all positive and he had absolute confidence in their veracity, how did he gain such insight to a psychotic state of mind to the extent of making madness a central theme of his poetic works, yet succeeded in maintaining his sanity?

The well-documented remark of Blake's wife that she had little communication with her husband as he was 'always in Paradise', suggests that his visionary experiences were, on the whole, ongoing, which may have applied to his youth and later life. Blake speaks, however, in a letter written in 1804 when he was 47, of his joy and relief that his 'visions' had returned to the positive intensity he had not known '... for twenty dark, but very profitable years. I thank God that I courageously pursued my course through darkness' (Keynes, 1979: 852). William James experienced a short period of darkness. For Carl Jung the severe depression, bordering on psychosis, lasted for seven years. To have suffered such agony intermittently over a period of 20 years, without falling into a state of madness, shows tremendous powers of endurance.

Blake mentions that despite the darkness, those years were 'profitable'. His published works, with some gaps, certainly span a period from 1769 to 1827, the year of his death. From childhood, the supernatural was a natural part of life for William Blake. Life-affirming contact with the world of spirit was his *raison d'être*. To have this positive contact withdrawn, particularly for such an extended period, would have left an agonizing void within his heart and mind. Is it possible that such darkness and suffering are necessary for the acquiring of deep insight into the meaning of human existence and that the greater the endurance, the greater the insight?

Blake's proximity to the mind/body split of madness is clarified by the following statement: 'I have indeed fought thro' a Hell of terrors & horrors (which none could know but myself) in a Divided Existence' (Keynes,

1979: 935). Was it by enduring such mental agony, with the support of his wife and the memory of his 'visions', that Blake was given access to the concept of madness without passing over the 'threshold', relieved to some extent by his ability to channel his experiences into creative pursuits?

The creative fields do offer an outlet for expression of personal perceptions: a necessity for 'suffering souls'. Van Gogh's paintings, for example, speak volumes to discerning viewers, and art collectors pay exorbitant prices to obtain his masterpieces; paintings produced by one with an unbalanced, demented mind whose keenly sensitive view of life and the universe penetrated way beyond normal human perceptions. Not all creative people are mentally disturbed of course (although it is a common feature among those involved in the arts), and many masterpieces and great literary works are produced by sane individuals. Does the unbalanced mind bring something special to its creations by reaching into a dimension inaccessible to others of more stable background and personality?

But what, you might ask, has all this to do with Grace and her spiritual journey? Suffice to say, she understood – to the limited degree anyone can understand the mind of another – the downward spiralling effects of depression and reported borderline experiences of the distinguished gentleman; to the forsaken effects of withdrawal of spiritual awareness; to the difficult role of faith (especially in oneself and one's judgement) while in the midst of inner turmoil. Why is it that for no apparent reason, or perhaps in reaction to a remark from another, the mind can suddenly switch over to a negative perception of what had a few seconds earlier been 'normal'? This tightrope existence of insecurity can become a living hell, as Grace discovered. Her reaction to these horrible feelings was depair and fear, fear being at the root of all mental illness; fear of life, fear of the future, fear of non-existence.

What on earth can be done for someone in such a desperate situation? For many, suicide seems the only way out; some manage to ride out the storm, while others lapse into psychosis. Fortunately for Grace, the spiritual connection made in childhood reactivated in response to a plea for help, but only after a period of preparation. Healing of painful wounds, sense of wholeness and freedom of spirit, with her puppet 'strings' disappearing, accompanied Grace's 'awakening' as the scattered jigsaw pieces of her mind suddenly fell into place, and heart and mind harmoniously connected.

Spiritual awakening

People of different religious persuasion make various interpretations of 'conversion' experiences. For instance, the 'mental catastrophe' of satori

– a state of sudden intuited Enlightenment, following the physical and mental disciplines practised by Zen Buddhists – relates to the Christian 'conversion' experience, with a 'new heaven' opening up for the perceiver. The concept of 'new birth', a feature of satori, is also that of the 'born again' Christian; as is a new perspective on life. The Bible records '... it is no longer I who live, but it is Christ who lives in me' (Gal. 2: 20) The converted Christian is given insight to a view of humanity and the natural world through the eyes, and with the mind, of Christ. William James records the reaction of one convert, which covers, in simple terms, the concept of 'new birth' and changed perception of the world: '... everything looked new to me, the people, the fields, the cattle, the trees. I was like a new man in a new world.' (James, 1982: 249).

The awakening of the spirit, judging from personal testimonies and altered outward behavioural patterns, can radically transform both the lifestyle of the experiencer and his or her perspective on life, suddenly or gradually. For many, the reality of everyday, normal existence on earth shifts to a reality that expands to produce a variety of new, previously unimagined concepts of life and the universe. The boundaries and limitations of human existence are claimed to have opened out, at least temporarily, exposing some of the wonders and offering glimpses of the mysteries lying behind the reality of the material world. With gradual or sudden removal of this veil, or awakening to the reality of the 'other' world, phenomena such as 'visions', 'voices' or 'presences' are frequently reported by experiencers. A significant feature of such experiences is the indelible impression made on the individual and often a sense of timelessness; of touching something of the eternal.

The files of the Alister Hardy Religious Experience Research Centre at Lampeter University, Wales, contain numerous modern reports of a variety of spiritual experiences.

Grace's initial experiences were of a religious nature, but other events, seemingly unrelated to spirituality, can 'convert' an individual's perspective on life. Being struck down by serious illness, an accident, grief at the loss of a loved one, or simply the ageing process usually results in a change of perception and outlook on life – sometimes for the better. Life can become more precious; a sense of rebirth or second chance may be experienced. Priorities are often readjusted as an understanding of what is really important in life comes into perspective. It is then, with the stripping away of secular, materialistic thought patterns, that spiritual awareness has the opportunity to filter through the mind and heart of the experiencer.

Following such life-fulfilling experiences, it would seem that Grace's spiritual journey had ended. The early spiritual 'seeds' planted in her young mind had at last germinated, blossoming into a vibrant bouquet of truth, as she reconnected with Donne's image of a human/Divine link – the spiritual link Grace had lost sight of as she went her own way, ignoring the good advice of her guiding conscience. 'Conversion', of course, was only a part – albeit the highlight – of her spiritual journey, and life continued to be a struggle in some respects, as unresolved relationship problems and physical illness took their toll. Her old negative personality, harbouring doubts about her own abilities when times were particularly difficult, persisted in rearing its ugly head – encouraged, she felt sure, by some forces determined, it seemed, to disrupt her life and destroy the spiritual progress she had made.

Spirituality and psychosis

As a consequence of her spiritual experiences and years of emotional turmoil, Grace became interested in the spiritual/psychotic relationship, discovering in RD Laing someone who understood the connection and really cared about the mentally distressed. She admired his courage in speaking out against the establishment in an effort to improve attitudes to, and treatments for, schizophrenic patients, becoming a powerful voice for those who are unable to speak coherently for themselves while in the throes of mental illness.

Grace realized how someone caught up in the psychiatric system, as a result of being overwhelmed by some dramatic, possibly negative, spiritual experience, could easily be diagnosed psychotic and prescribed the standard drug treatment programme if details of the experience were disclosed; especially if the hearer rejected the concept of spirituality. How would a sceptical psychiatrist respond, for example, if told by a patient: 'While preparing dinner one evening, moving between the kitchen and dining room, a voice – in my head – said quite distinctly, "Sit down and listen, this is important". I realized the command was to pay attention to the person being interviewed on television and I sat and watched the news item.'? What if the patient claimed to have experienced an awesome vision of God, so powerful the mind's eye had to be closed against it? Grace was very relieved she had never been drawn into the psychiatric system.

Criticism of RD Laing (who died in 1989) and his writings continues to this day. But articles in modern mental health publications reveal that the concerns of Ronald Laing – such as the sane/mad, doctor/patient divide, suppressive treatment and power of psychiatrists over patients – are still being criticized by those caught up in the psychiatric system. Pleas are made to consider the life histories of mental health patients, rather than merely clinical analyses, which further isolate the patient, ruling out attempts to make personal contact. Writers suggest looking into reasons for the abnormal behaviour of schizophrenic patients and attempting to remove the influences that cause such behaviour, rather than dampening the symptoms with drugs. The crucial effects of a personality interacting with the environment and the need for caring, nurturing responses from care workers are other views expressed.

Conclusion

I began by defining spirituality in contrast to materialism. William Blake accepted that his spiritual perceptions differed from the 'material hell' of others, and Erskine and James, with their own interpretations, placed the onus on each individual to choose between the two. Erskine's theory that the conscience is the centre of spiritual truth suggests that the advice from Jiminy Cricket was good grounding for life in the Spirit; as was the moral code of religious teaching. For someone with Grace's sensitive, vulnerable personality, however, emphasis on constraining religious commands, rather than freely given, unconditional love, created a guilt complex and consequent emotional and relationship problems.

It was argued that spirituality cannot be experienced by rational means, enabling young children and the simple minded to be blessed with spiritual awareness, though many of the materially minded, worldly successful appear to lead happy lives. Kierkegaard claims, however, that the most favoured dwelling place for despair is '... deep in the heart of happiness' (Kierkegaard, 1989: 55) – a warning not to be motivated by a manufactured 'false' self to the neglect of a self made in the image of God, the 'true' self. But to choose life in the Spirit is generally regarded in today's world as weakness, folly, even insanity, so why make such a choice?

Grace's experiences in her early contact with Donne's concept of a human/divine link, and later reawakening, illustrate some of the problems encountered in adopting a 'false' self and ignoring the spiritual truths addressed to the conscience. As Jung's introvert personality no doubt increased his negative reaction to the break with Freud, so Grace's difficulties in coping with the problems inevitably occurring during life's journey arose mainly from her sensitive nature. Conversely, Blake's tempestuous temperament enabled him to remain indifferent to the responses of others, but the withdrawal of his affirming 'visions' left him vulnerable to negative forces and led to his 'threshold' experiences, which, it was suggested, may be necessary to gain deep insight into the meaning of life. Would Jung and Blake, for example, have found the ability to create their important testimonies to spiritual truth without both the ecstasy and agony they experienced?

Unlike the restrained reaction to her childhood experience, following the initial adult experiences Grace felt overwhelmingly compelled to reach out to others, to share with them her newfound knowledge in the hope of alleviating at least some of the sorrow and misunderstanding in the world. Her Christian background enabled Grace to find a framework for interpretation of the experiences – or it seems more likely they were created in an appropriate form for her particular needs – and she was led to hearers who generally responded positively to what was revealed. Grace believes, however, that had the adult experiences or her reactions been negative and she had subsequently sought psychiatric help, and if hearers had responded with dismissal or rejection of her reports, she would undoubtedly have 'gone under'.

The excruciatingly painful open wound of a tortured mind is unbearably sensitive to the touch. If hearers dismiss reports of other-world experiences simply as 'unreal' or refuse to listen with an open mind to such reports, the wound receives further untold injury and trauma by introducing doubts, conflict, and frustration, tipping the finely balanced scales of the unstable mind on a downward path. RD Laing defines the schizophrenic sufferer as, literally, '... one who is broken hearted (schizo – "broken", Phrenos – "soul" or "heart") and even broken hearts have been known to mend, if we have the heart to let them' (Laing, 1967: 107). Please, for all in mental or emotional agony, let's find the heart.

References

Hanna W (1878) Letters of Thomas Erskine of Linlathen, 3rd edn. Edinburgh: David Douglas.

Hardy A (1978) The Divine Flame. Oxford: RERC reprint.

Hardy A (1997) The Spiritual Nature of Man. Oxford: RERC reprint.

Hay D (1998) The Spirit of the Child. London: HarperCollins.

Jackson M (1991) A study of the relationship between psychotic and spiritual experience. DPhil thesis, Trinity College, Dublin.

James W (1982) The Varieties of Religious Experience. NJ: Penguin.

Jung CG (1983) Memories, Dreams, Reflections. London: Fontana.

Keynes G (ed.) (1979) Blake: complete writings. Oxford: Oxford University Press.

Kierkegaard S (1989) The Sickness Unto Death. London: Penguin.

Laing, RD (1967) The Politics of Experience and The Bird of Paradise. Harmondsworth: Penguin.

Youngquist P (1989) Madness and Blake's Myth. Pennsylvania State University.

Chapter 4

Climbing Dürer's Ladder[1]

PHIL BARKER AND POPPY BUCHANAN-BARKER

Some altered states

The boy's own story

His wife lay silently beside him as the room slowly darkened. He watched the shadows forming and knew that he was not entering *Shadowland* but was trapped in no-man's-land. He sensed the width of his internal ocean, balancing himself on a paper-thin edge, where notions of sensation held no currency. As his hand moved across his chest he felt the silver dust on his body, wondering – momentarily – how he could *feel* a colour, like silver. His chest had an alien solidity, almost denying its organic function. It felt solid yet waxen. Indeed, his body was made of wax, upon which was sprinkled silver dust: no ordinary dust, but dust that registered its silver-like appearance through touch.

He drew a deep breath and his waxen frame moved without disturbing its angelic coating. With each inspiration the dimensions of the room stretched to ludicrous proportions and he watched, dispassionately, as the small window, which let in the sky, retreated, pulling the perspective of everything in the room with it. He had been here so many times before over the past decade that he almost apologized for asking, again, if he was awake or dreaming. He roused his waxen frame, noting that he felt here and 'not here' at one and the same moment. The first time he had tried to rise up out of that strange state, he was only just stepping out of childhood. In that first simple rising he found himself questioning the nature of reality. More than ten years later, he knew that this was not a simple

---

[1] This chapter draws on a paper presented at the Consultation on Spirituality, held in St George's House, Windsor Castle, England, on 5 December 1998.

question, or even just a complex one. It was a question which might well be ineffable. He was not sure that he knew what *ineffable* meant but, in that moment, the meaning visited him again, and he felt the awesomeness of nothing coursing silently through his waxen body, framed within the ridiculous perspective of the room. He knew that this experience would not be limited to this small room. He knew that he would meet the great ineffable in other parts of his perceptual world. There, as here, his senses of touch and perception would belittle him, and he would wait patiently, as he had done before, until they returned him to what he understood to be Reality, or not.

He appeared to be in a class, perhaps of his own, perhaps even a class of his own making; but certainly he was receiving instruction. 'God help me,' he murmured quietly to himself, 'if I know what I am being taught, far less what I am learning.'

The girl's own story

She could only have been seven or eight when she began having a very vivid, recurring dream. A battle was taking place in the field behind her house. The field was well known to her as she had been born in this house and used the field daily as a playground. In the dream it was transformed into a battlefield from a distant but vivid past. It was hand-to-hand combat with fighting men on foot and there was smoke everywhere. She would always see the same scene and then would find herself in another part of the house with her older brother, when through the window would climb one of the soldiers from the battle.

This was the point at which she always woke up.

The dream seemed to be fixed in her memory and she never told anyone about it until she was in her late teens. Now that she is older, she is aware that although she has not had the dream for many years, any memory of it still makes her feel vaguely unsettled.

One day, by chance, she discovered that a battle had taken place very near the field at the back of her house. She was intrigued to learn that 200 of the men who had taken part, all of whom died, were from the Clan Buchanan and the date of the battle was around 17 July 1651. Her birthday is 17 July and her family name is Buchanan.

Translating the story of the self

Increasingly, neuroscience encourages us to believe that we know how the brain creates the mind, if not also the person. These assumptions carry the implication that human experience is meaningless – no more than the waste products of a brain that is constantly inventing and reinventing itself. In medicine, the psychiatric knowledge base has shifted within less than 50 years from the assumption that the many variants of the human personality are largely a function of lived experience, to the assumption that the *mind* is largely a function (distantly) of genetic influence and (more proximally) of biological gurgling. The best known of the neo-Darwinians, Richard Dawkins, has argued that human life is no more than a function of "'a concatenation of inane events whose only connecting thread is the propagation and survival of limited structure-carrying systems such as genes", a bleak view of the meaningless character of life on earth' (quoted in Polkinghorne, 1996: 1).

We are also encouraged to take the view that the *content*, which makes up the experience of psychosis, is similarly meaningless; the mere outcome of one neurophysiological anomaly or another. This may make laboratory sense, but doesn't travel well in the social world of experience. Some people described as 'suffering from schizophrenia' report hearing voices that tell them to lead the world to God or, as in the case of the blues musician Peter Green, to give away all their money. Others hear voices urging them to kill people or, as in the case of Peter Sutcliffe – the infamous Yorkshire Ripper – to kill *only* women. As Boyle (1990) has observed, if these people are 'ailing' from something, they have very different ailments indeed. The idea that these very different ways of 'being in the world' stem from a neurophysiological anomaly seems even more far fetched than the traditional notion that such people are possessed by demons.

No less an authority than Francis Crick, who was part of the team that unravelled the mystery of DNA, has sought to collapse all subtle distinctions among the mad, bad and dangerous to know, with a reductionist scenario that includes even those who consider themselves to be 'sane', whatever that might mean, with his assertion that:

> You – your joys and your sorrows, your memories and your ambitions, your sense of personal identity and free will – are in fact no more than the behaviour of a vast assembly of nerve cells and their associated molecules.

> Crick (1994: 4)

This view of the *mind* gives rise to a few problems, as Polkinghorne, the particle physicist has noted:

> At the material pole of reality, if you split me apart into my constituents, you will just find quarks and gluons and electrons. You will also have destroyed me. The self resides at the other, holistic, pole of reality. That explains its elusiveness in the reductive analyses of materialism or computer functionalism ... signs that one is looking in the wrong place, scrabbling around among the pieces for what can only be found in the whole.

> Polkinghorne (1996: 72)

Crick, and many other contemporary neuroscientists, are suggesting that this is, in Crick's famous phrase, an *astonishing hypothesis*. In Szasz's view, nothing could be further from the truth – it is simply an echo of Hippocrates' view that the mind is a function of the brain: 'a facile equation that never lost its appeal' (Szasz, 1996: 84).

Although we talk glibly now about mental *health* services, at their heart lies a great and powerful rush to reframe all human experience within the terrorism of *normality*: human death by psychiatric diagnosis.

Dissenting voices

Although whole generations of people have been colonized and forced into submission by crude systems of 'psychiatric care' (Whitaker, 2001), a new wave of dissent has emerged over the past decade. In particular, the dissenting voices of people who have been redefined by psychiatric diagnosis have recently grown to a clamour. We would like to introduce some truly expert witnesses: people who have journeyed to the furthest reaches of their own human nature and returned to tell the tale of madness and its possible spiritual undercurrents.

Sally's story

Sally Clay was a student at an American college when she discovered, 'like other mad people [her words] ... mental states that transformed my mind but also shattered my world ... What others of my generation explored with psychedelic drugs, I discovered through a natural explosion of thoughts and emotions. Sitting alone in a small dormitory room I journeyed into the depths of the mind and the heights of the universe. I found in everyday objects the essence of atoms, and in the familiarity of stars the basis of quantum physics. In a flash of passion I understood the interdependence of all events and the unity of all spirit. I glimpsed a truth more real than anything else I had known and achieved a transformation of mind that was lasting. This altered state was both my exaltation and my downfall' (Clay, 1999).

Unlike the synthetic drug experience, the effect of this breakthrough to a higher consciousness did not wear off. Sally gradually lost touch with everyday life as both new and old realities were swept from beneath her. She underwent many years of crude psychiatric intervention masquerading as treatment, sitting, as she noted 'day after day among blank-faced men and women lined up in their chaise-longues around the sides of the glassed-in porch of limbo-land'.

Here, Sally discovered the almost universal psychiatric truth: that recovery is synonymous with the erasure of any individual beliefs or hopes except those standardized by society and represented through the authority of her psychiatrist. Here she came to believe that if there was any meaning in the world, it was known only to her psychiatrist and his nurses, and if known by the rest of the world it had been forever lost her. She noted, 'I had not lost just my education and my future but even my soul.'

When Sally looked back down the 30 years of her career in madness she could identify certain staging posts in her recovery:

> Several of us in the 'recovered' category have described our extreme mental states in the hope that these might inspire examination of what really happens in the mind, as well as the body of the person labelled mentally ill. If we are recovered, what is it that we have recovered from? If we are well now and were sick before, what is it that we have recovered to? For some reason the dialogue never gets off the ground. The psychiatrists become visibly uneasy when the subject arises and they divert the discussion to a less threatening thought. 'Coping mechanisms' are just such a diversion, an attempt to regard the depth of madness as something that can be simply 'coped' with.
>
> Clay (1999)

Sally eventually found psychiatric rescue in Ed Podvoll, the Buddhist-inspired psychiatrist, who became her therapist, and then encouraged her to become a 'wounded healer'. Reflecting on Ed's hypothesis about the *Seduction of Madness* (Podvoll, 1990), Sally noted that:

> What is so compelling about madness is the tantalising hint that it holds the secrets of consciousness, of healing, and spiritual power. It is madness that brings our attention to the mind, that makes us remember that mind is inseparable from spirit, that it is consciousness that makes us human.
>
> Clay (1999)

Cathy's story

Our Australian friend Cathy Conroy has drawn attention to psychiatry's failure to address the richness of the experience of madness:

> Breakdown, the first time, contains rich and strong spiritual memories. The remnants of these memories form a pattern, as if from an inner weaving, a carpeted mandala. The richness of the textual design is not often discussed in mental health services. Most of the psychiatrists I have encountered while a mental health advocate have spent virtually no time on the *substance* of the mentally ill person's experience, its potential in working towards the development of inner emotional and spiritual connections.
>
> Conroy (1999)

Reflecting on her own breakdowns, Cathy recalled that:

> Collage was an important part of my recovery. It seemed to offer me clarity, as I ripped pictures from magazines, assembling the fragments of photos and illustrations in a way that encapsulated my inner experience. The fragments formed symbols of my psychic world, emerging from the depths of inner caverns. The meanings I attributed have remained very important to me in understanding the patterns in my life contributing to my health and my illness.
>
> Conroy (1999)

Touching meaningfulness

Both Sally and Cathy show that madness has a function and that part of that function is to reveal meaning in life (Frankl, 1964), but perhaps also meaning beyond the limits of life (Frankl, 2000). Cathy Conroy recognized the value of waiting, which, as Mathew Fox has said, is for most of us an uncomfortable thing to do. However, when we settle down to it, we realize that it is a deep part of the whole spiritual process (Fox, 1991: 4). Cathy saw her path stretching 'through long cold months of painful loss of feeling, awaiting the season of shooting buds on a swelling heart, to melt the snow and ice'.

She believed that her heartache is best summed up in the words of George Steiner:

> We are haunted by the sense of a breach with the promise in ourselves, with the best possibilities within ourselves. That hauntedness perhaps is our guilt.
>
> Conroy (1999)

The poetics of Cathy Conroy's waiting game appear to have brought her closer to a true notion of wholeness and health and appear to have healed her own breach of promise. Meanwhile psychiatry continues to grapple, dualistically, with madness as *illness*, appearing only to drive the wedge of false rationality further between the *I* and the *me* of experience. For Sally Clay the question remained:

> If mental illness is a disease of the mind, what is the nature of the mind? If altered states have value, what is there to recover from? What is our model of wellness? Is it true as some say, that our spiritual realization is the highest aspiration of the human race? If it is, should not that be our model of wellness? How do we recover to that state of wellness?
>
> Clay (1999)

Psychiatry maintains the view that people who commune with gods, angels and other spirits are, in the main, broken, unstable and unworthy communicants. The ever-increasing narrowness of psychiatric vision blinds us to the sociological, anthropological and historical facts that people have been communing in much the same kind of way with spirits for as long as we have been able to record such stories. Sally begs the questions:

> Why do people in mania consistently experience an urgent call to save the world, and call themselves messiah or saviour? Is this merely grandiose, or do such people truly hear a call to help others?

> Why in this culture are some forms of mental illness so excruciatingly painful and so interminable? Is the reason illness, or is there a tragic mis-understanding of global proportions? Who is ill – is it the visionary or is it the society itself?

Clay (1999)

The thread of understanding

Some connections are being made here that are worth noting. Sally Clay was mentored by Ed Podvoll who, in turn, was mentored by Ronnie Laing among others. More than 30 years ago Laing reopened the debate about the spiritual dimension of madness and, like Sally, questioned who exactly was the madder – the patient or the society that requested the confine-ment of the patient. Thirty years on, Laing is dismissed as a reckless and unbalanced iconoclast, and like other pioneers of the psychotic journey before him, Harry Stack Sullivan and Carl Jung, questions are asked about his mental stability (Barker and Buchanan-Barker, 2002). This prompts us to ask:

- What is normal?
- What is the true nature of reality?
- Most importantly, what is the nature and value of suffering?

Cathy Conroy reflected on her continuing struggle with madness and found solace in Ken Wilber, who said:

> A person who is beginning to sense the suffering of life is, at the same time, beginning to awaken deeper realities, truer realities. For suffering smashes to pieces the complacency of our normal fictions about reality, and forces us to become alive in a special sense – to see carefully, to feel deeply, to touch ourselves and our worlds in ways we have heretofore avoided ... suf-fering is the first grace. In a special sense, suffering is almost a time of rejoic-ing, for it marks the birth of creative insight.

Wilber (1985)

The mad psychiatrist

Our third witness is our colleague Dan Fisher, who experienced a schizo-phrenic psychosis when a research scientist in his early twenties. He is now a community psychiatrist, and Director of the National Empowerment Center in Massachusetts. Talking about recovery Dan noted:

> I no longer search for the sickness in myself or in those I grew up with as an explanation for my woes. Instead I search for the strengths in myself, and those close to me, which propel me through my version of the suffering we all share but seldom face. I, psychiatry and our society need to shift away from our current perspective, featuring negative feedback and a pathologi-cal emphasis on *external locus of control*; we should shift toward a person-driven, democratic *internal locus of control* perspective.
>
> Fisher (1999)

Regrettably, the popular political and professional emphases remain on externality and the myth of the mind in the brain, with a virtual dis-appearance of the person within and beyond the mind. Dan Fisher is, however, one of a small, yet growing number of psychiatrists (cf. Culliford, 2002) who are locating spirit at the core of their survival. Dan writes of the essential aspects of recovery:

> There is inside of me a self, a spirit, which is gradually becoming more aware of me and others. That self is becoming my guide. It encompasses all that I am. My self includes, but is greater than, my chemicals, my back-ground and my traumas: it is the me I am seeking to become in my rela-tionships in that moment of creative uncertainty when I make contact with another. From that moment of harmony, when, together, we defy the odds and say 'yes', our lives will go on differently, regardless of how we live the following moment. We are all inventing our lives at each moment.

Beyond flatland

Dan Fisher draws our attention to a simple, yet paradoxical point: our psychological selves encompass our biological and biochemical selves, and our psychological selves are bounded by our spiritual selves. The 'I' that is 'me' is part of *me*, but is greater than me alone. Similarly, the per-sonal 'me' is part of the material 'me' but is greater than 'me' alone. The blinkering effect of scientific empiricism has led to a denial of the evident truth of the great 'nest of being' we have hinted at here, where even the most microscopic aspect of being 'me' lies nestled within increasingly greater aspects of being until we find our 'selves' in the being of the cosmos. As Wilber has noted:

> There has been in the West, for the last three hundred years or so, a profound and aggressive attempt by modern science, to completely reduce the entire Kosmos to a bunch of 'its'. That is the I and we domains have been almost entirely colonized by the it-domains, by scientific materialism, positivism, behaviorism, empiricism, and objective-exterior approaches in general.
>
> Wilber (1998: 21)

This is the great project of subtle *reductionism*.

> Mind is reduced to brain; praxis is reduced to techne; interiors are reduced to bits of digital its; depth is reduced to endless surfaces roaming a flat and faded system; levels of quality are reduced to levels of quantity; dialogical interpretation is reduced to monological gaze – in short, the multidimensional universe is rudely reduced to flatland.
>
> Wilber (1997: 21)

Although contemporary psychiatry and psychology pretends to be 'holistic', with its genuflection before notions of systems theory, cybernetic feedback mechanisms, complexity and chaos theory, and the like, it continues to reduce all 'I's and all 'we's to info-its, as Wilber said:

> ... running through neuronal it-pathways carried by it-neurotransmitters to it-goals. Your presence, your existence, your consciousness is not required. That these are often holistic and systems-oriented approaches is no solace at all: that's simply subtle reductionism at its worst: a flatland web of interwoven its.
>
> Wilber (1997: 22–23)

We have opted instead to define the interior experience by what science assumes to be its exterior form. Paradoxically, what for the behavioural scientist lies on the *outside* of our experience – the behaviour of our muscles and molecules – in truth lies inside of our mind, which in turn lies within our souls, which is ultimately nestled within spirit, which encompasses everything – ourselves and the world of experience.

This conceptualization, which is ancient, has been lost in our search to ground our knowledge in verifiable, concrete reality – materialism. This 'flatland' of postmodern science has led to the diminishment of the importance of art and morals and contemplation and spirit, all of which have been demolished by what Wilber calls 'the scientific bull in the china shop of consciousness'.

Flatland began with the Enlightenment, and escalates today in the neuroscientific redefinition of personhood as chemistry. Ironically, the neuroscientists find support among the postmodern philosophers of deconstruction, who also reduce everything to the flattest surface: there is no within – surface, surface, surface is all. Of course, if there is only surface, if language or chemicals define everything – even within systems theory, chaos theory or complexity – where can we find anything resembling beauty, poetry, creative expression, value, desire, love, honour, moral wisdom, compassion or charity, far less God or the Goddess?

The stories, which we have drawn from our witnesses, challenge this flatland mentality. The altered states found in most forms of madness may have biological correlates, but their inherent complexity of content has never been explained by biological psychiatry. The eminent psychiatrist and psychopharmacologist David Healy has noted that:

> One strong indication that hallucinations result from fevers of the psyche rather than of the brain is that the perceptions involved are not just any perceptions as one might expect from abnormal brain function ... To have detailed and complex hallucinations probably *requires* one's brain to be functioning normally ... a prerequisite of complex hallucinations is an altered psychological state rather than an altered brain state.

> Healy (1990: 163–165)

Healy's emphasis on altered states echoes our witnesses and finds an older echo in William James, who, after many years of study of the varieties of human experience, concluded:

> Our normal waking consciousness, rational consciousness as we call it, is but one special type of consciousness, whilst all about it, parted from it by the flimsiest of screens, there lie potential forms of consciousness entirely different. We may go through life without suspecting their existence; but apply the requisite stimulus, and at a touch they are there in all their completeness.

> James (1902: 378)

Dürer's ladder

Albrecht Dürer offered the most famous, and arguably the most misunderstood, image of *melancholia*, historically the commonest form of madness. The winged figure of Melancholia, in Dürer's famous engraving, sits immobilized by sorrow, her head resting on a clenched fist, eyes fixed in a glassy stare. Her hair and clothing is manifestly dishevelled. She is surrounded by the symbols and tools of the creative process but appears to be suffering from what Panofsky called the 'tragic unrest of human creation' (Panofsky, 1955). She appears destined, in her paradoxical union of genius and despair, to lose her competition with God, the ultimate creator. This is commonly seen as the spiritual self-portrait of Dürer, who was inspired by celestial influences and eternal ideas, but who suffered all the more deeply when he failed to climb the ladder – depicted in the background of the image – which would allow him to transcend the human condition. This is the received view of Dürer's most enigmatic work (cf. Schildkraut and Otero, 1996).

We offer an alternative interpretation. Rather than being debilitated by depression, Dürer recognized this state as a superior form of melancholy, characteristic of thinkers and artists. Rather than an image of despair and bottomless sadness, Dürer's engraving suggests *inspired listening, sensitivity* to the *mysterious language of the imagination*, compared with which the instruments and other pieces of scientific apparatus which litter the scene are of little importance (cf. Barker, 1992; Knappe, 1965). The angel – who bears a striking resemblance to Dürer himself – gazes upon various mathematical tools, strewn on the ground before her. Dürer was fascinated by the mathematics of ratio, and for some time believed that he might be able to compose the perfect image, with ratio's help. The melancholic figure appears to represent the momentary realization that this was a tragically false, inflated and, of course, unnecessary ambition. Vanity reaps its own reward and her name is rejection.

From this perspective the image may be read as a challenge to materialism and all other 'false gods' that might serve as diversions from the chosen path (enlightenment), symbolized by the ladder, which stands against a wall in the background. This is the metaphorical means by which it will be possible to be connected to a higher plane of existence in this world, rather than a means of escape into the next.

In the context of our contemporary 'scientific' world view, the ladder also possesses great significance. As Polkinghorne (1996) has noted, if we 'descend' deeper and deeper into the physical, material reality of ourselves, we shall eventually descend into nothingness. We are all aware that the firm body we feel, whether muscular or fat, is composed, in the main, of water. Our sheer physicality is sensory illusion. In the story of physics the illusion is far more intimidating. If we journey through the tissue, to the cellular level and press on beyond the atomic and subatomic levels of our 'being', ultimately we shall emerge into nothingness. Or perhaps, we shall find ourselves back where we entered this story – in the wider frame of reference of the cosmos.

Dürer's ladder may be read as a metaphor for the route of ascension to a higher plane of understanding – if not within the cosmos, at least within this material realm of reality. The ladder, however, like many perennial truths, embraces a paradox. As we climb to each rung of the ladder, we move closer to the absolute totality of God or the Spirit or – as the physicists might say, the explanation of everything. In one sense, Spirit is the summit of all being. This is the ultimate soul, of which we all seek to be a part. Spirit, or soul, is the highest rung on the ladder of evolution. However, Spirit is also the wood out of which the entire ladder and all of its rungs are made. 'Spirit is the suchness, the isness and the essence of everything that exists' (Wilber, 1997: 44). So, while we appear to 'journey' towards God, in search of the absolute, in pursuit of our spiritual selves, seeking salvation for our souls, the spiritual revelation we seek is already here, echoing the Chinese saying, 'the journey of a thousand miles begins under your very feet'. As we set out in search of the Path of Enlightenment, we are already on the Path. As Chödrön said, 'start where you are' (Chödrön, 1994). Or, as the Celtic visionaries noted, the journey out in search of everything, always ends back at home.

Our witnesses help us to sober up, in a sense. Mental health has, invariably, been defined as being, in a very basic sense, 'in touch with reality'. As we have noted, if we turn to the hardest of sciences – nuclear physics – to determine the nature of such 'bedrock reality', we find that there is nothing there. As Wilber noted, we are just as likely to be told by the physicists, as by the religious zealot, that 'reality actually exists in the mind of some eternal spirit'. If we find this too absurd, too unreal, then who are we to believe? If sanity is the goal then, as Wilber asked (Wilber, 1997: 2), 'exactly what reality are we supposed to be in touch with?

The future is now *and* in the past

The common assumption that there exists a simple boundary line between the 'sane' and the 'mad' is one of the prevailing delusions of the postmodern age. The evidence that can be found, especially in the lives of creative people, is that creativity and madness often overlap (Pickering, 1974; Schildkraut and Otero, 1996). It seems more likely that all sorts of people stray across this imaginary boundary at one time or another in their lives, stepping from our assumptions of a bounded and material universe into something reaching into the beyond (Barker, 1996; Wilber, 1985).

To conclude, we return to our opening stories. The boy's story was – and in an important sense, remains – Phil's story. The decade-long chain of experiences, which ended as abruptly as they had begun, prompted him to become interested in his own consciousness and that of others: to begin asking 'Who am I? What am I? Why am I?' He learned, as countless others had learned before him, that our feelings, thoughts, impulses, images and other related human sensations are the contents of our consciousness; the witnesses that we *are*. However, in the context of *how* these experiences are experienced, the 'I' of consciousness lies in awareness of such phenemona. We *know* we are here, because *we* experience 'here'. However, as Alan Watts would have observed, when I say that I am aware, who is the 'I' that is aware that I am aware? What is the 'radical self' that is the source of the manifest world and that was *known* by the ancients?

In denial of such wisdom, we have assumed for generations that a person who experiences depression is depressed *and* (ergo) 'a depressive'. Deikman (1996) has helped us appreciate that 'I *am* awareness'. 'I *know* I *am* by *being* "I"' (awareness). Regrettably, few people appear to have the experience of helping professionals, like Deikman, to help them toward the experience of 'I' as 'awareness'. Instead, we appear compelled to encourage people to believe that *they* are a by-product of their biochemistry, or even an organic pathology. Hence, the continued *colonization* of so many people to admit to *being* schizophrenics, manic depressives or alcoholics, instead of being in *awareness* of being *in* states of being that society, temporarily, refers to as schizophrenia, etc.

The girl's story was Poppy's story. When she first discovered the details of the actual battle, and pieced together the facts of what had taken place, she felt shocked yet strangely elated. In a sense, she felt connected strongly to the past and her ancestors. It led her to believe that her dream represented a way for the spirits of the past to live on. It also led her to think about the lives of people who had gone before her and the fact that the land was so important for them that they would march hundreds of miles on foot, many of them to almost certain death. However, since she found out about the battle, she has had much more difficulty in recalling the details of her dream, which she had carried around with her for almost 40 years. It was almost as if the connection had been made and the dream was no longer necessary.

She feels very privileged to be so connected to these brave people and to call them her ancestors. She believes that it is from them that she gains her emotional strength, and her motto has long been, 'always march to the sound of gunfire'.

The childhood stories of Phil and Poppy have become part of the emerging story of their adult lives. They lie nestled within their later experiences, which lie in wait for the next set of experiences, which will wrap around them, like a new covering of bark on a tree. Like the tree, we grow outwards into the world, but draw our strength from the core of our being, which lies rooted in the soil, which in turn draws its strength from the whole planet, which lies nestled within the cosmos.

With such metaphors we might build a bridge between the wisdom of the ancients and the soul of contemporary physics and cosmology. Eddie Kneebone, an Aboriginal educator, provided an echo of Poppy's appreciation for the land of her ancestors and the spiritual connections that were passed through her in her 'dreamtime', when he defined:

Aboriginal spirituality is the belief and the feeling within yourself that allows you to become part of the whole environment around you – not the built environment, but the natural environment ... Birth, life and death are all part of it, and you welcome each.

Kneebone (1991)

The soul or spirit will continue on after death of the physical form has passed away, and as Eddie said:

The spirit will return to the Dreamtime from where it came, it will carry out memories to the Dreamtime and eventually will return again through birth, either as human, animal or even trees or rocks. The shape is not important because everything is equal and shares the same soul or spirit from the Dreamtime.

Eddie Kneebone offers us a fitting conclusion by allowing us to ask whether we have forgotten that what inhabits us, ultimately, has no shape, is nothing, and is what unites us. We believe that Sally and Cathy and Dan all were thrown, violently, into their own witness of that radical self-hood, their place within the Great Nest of being and upon which rung they stood on Dürer's ladder. We feel that our introduction to our spiritual selves has been much gentler. For that we shall be, quite literally, eternally grateful.

References

Barker P (1992) Severe Depression: a practitioner's guide. London: Chapman and Hall.

Barker P (1996) Chaos and the way of Zen: psychiatric nursing and the 'uncertainty principle'. Journal of Psychiatric and Mental Health Nursing 3: 235–244.

Barker P and Buchanan-Barker P (2002) Medicine's turbulent priest. Openmind 116: 10–11.

Boyle M (1990) Schizophrenia: a scientific delusion? London: Routledge.

Chödrön P (1994) Start Where You Are: a guide to compassionate living. London: Shambhala.

Clay S (1999) Madness and reality. In: Barker P, Campbell P and Davidson B (eds) From the Ashes of Experience: reflections on madness, survival and growth. London: Whurr.

Conroy C (1999) Fire and ice. In: Barker P, Campbell P and Davidson B (eds) From the Ashes of Experience: reflections on madness, survival and growth. London: Whurr.

Crick F (1994) The Astonishing Hypothesis. New York: Simon and Schuster.

Culliford L (2002) Spiritual care and psychiatric treatment: an introduction. Advances in Psychiatric Treatment 8: 249–261.

Deikman AJ (1996) 'I' = awareness. Journal of Consciousness Studies 3: 350–356.

Fisher D (1999) Hope, humanity and voice in recovery from mental illness. In: Barker P, Campbell P and Davidson B (eds) From the Ashes of Experience: reflections on madness, survival and growth. London: Whurr.

Fox M (1991) Creation spirituality and the dreamtime. In: Hammond C (ed.) Creation Spirituality and the Dreamtime. Newtown, NSW: Millennium Books.

Frankl V (1964) Man's Search for Meaning. London: Hodder and Stoughton.

Frankl V (2000) Man's Search for Ultimate Meaning. Cambridge, MA: Perseus Publishing.

Healy D (1990) The Suspended Revolution. London: Faber.

James W (1902) The Varieties of Religious Experience. New York: Longmans Green.

Knappe KA (1965) Dürer: the complete engravings, etchings and woodcuts. London: Thames and Hudson.

Kneebone E (1991) An aboriginal response. In: Hammond C (ed.) Creation Spirituality and the Dreamtime. Newtown, NSW: Millennium Books.

Panofsky E (1955) The Life and Art of Albrecht Dürer. Princeton, NJ: Princeton University Press.

Pickering G (1974) Creative Malady: illness in the lives and minds of Charles Darwin, Florence Nightingale, Mary Baker Eddy, Sigmund Freud, Marcel Proust, Elizabeth Barrett Browning. London: George Allen and Unwin.

Podvoll E (1990) The Seduction of Madness. London: Century.

Polkinghorne J (1996) Beyond Science: the wider human context. Cambridge: Cambridge University Press.

Schildkraut JJ and Otero A (1996) Depression and the Spiritual in Modern Art: homage to Miró. Chichester: John Wiley and Sons.

Szasz TS (1996) The Meaning of Mind: language, morality and neuroscience. Westport and London: Praeger.

Whitaker R (2001) Mad in America. Bad science, bad medicine and the enduring mistreatment of the mentally ill. Cambridge, MA: Perseus Publishing.

Wilber K (1985) No Boundary. London: Shambhala.

Wilber K (1997) The Eye of the Spirit: an integral vision for a world gone slightly mad. London: Shambhala.

CHAPTER 5

A *Via Negativa* in the City: reflections from Whitechapel Road

KENNETH LEECH

Kenneth Leech is an Anglican priest who has been working in the East End of London for most of the time since 1958. He is the author of *Through Our Long Exile: contextual theology and the urban experience* and other books.

An Anglican Zen story

The late Archbishop Michael Ramsey was guest at a dinner for Anglican clergy and was placed next to the wife of one of them, a distinguished analytical psychologist. Ramsey had no small talk, and the following dialogue occurred after 15 minutes of silence.

Ramsey: What ... what do you do?

'Mary': I am a Jungian analyst.

Ramsey: Oh! Yes!

[Pause of five minutes]

Ramsey: Do you think that the dark night of the soul is the same thing as endogenous depression?

'Mary': No, I don't.

[Pause of three minutes]

Ramsey: Good. Good. Neither do I.

(For a slightly different version see De-la-Noy, 1990: 94)

There are things that can only be seen in darkened skies, questions only heard in the silence of utter dismay. Such a time is ours.

Ecclestone (1980: 39)

It was a common concern about homelessness that brought David Brandon and myself together in 1964. David had been appointed deputy superintendent of the London County Council's Welfare Centre for the Homeless at Charing Cross ('underneath the arches'). I was a newly ordained curate in Shoreditch, and, after several years of working with older homeless men, including methylated spirit drinkers – in Whitechapel, I was becoming increasingly involved with young amphetamine and intravenous heroin and cocaine users in the Shoreditch, Whitechapel and Bethnal Green districts of East London. David and I found common ground practically, academically and spiritually.

Not least, we shared the experience of being overwhelmed, swamped and 'brought down' by the sheer pressure of individual demands and needs. There were many occasions when work with homeless people and addicts brought us to a point of helplessness, hopelessness and spiritual exhaustion. It was a point close to despair, and yet there was something in that moment which inspired, nourished and strengthened us. As a Christian priest, nurtured in the tradition of Catholic spirituality, I was aware, at least – and for some time only – intellectually, of the emphasis by the mystics on 'unknowing' and on the creative potential of darkness. David, at that time a Quaker, was moving towards Zen Buddhism, with its focus on 'the void'. We found common ground in an approach to darkness which promised and provoked more than desolation of spirit.

A person who was a friend to, and influence on, both of us in those early years was the social worker Norman Ingram-Smith. In evidence given to a London County Council report on crude-spirit drinkers in 1964, he captured well the situation which we knew:

> Unwashed, evil smelling, incapable of work, occasionally emerging from his psychotic drunken state when restrained by the law or on an observation ward, he fights his bosom pal, he risks death by burning in disused houses. He is repulsive not only to others but to himself. Largely due to the aroma of his urine, he is unacceptable both in lodging houses and indeed in police cells. During the winter this kind of man spends his time in bombed out houses, under railway arches, in disused cars, and is frequently the victim of malnutrition, bronchitis and other diseases of deprivation and exposure. His condition gives rise to contempt even amongst the worst of the alcoholics who only drink recognised alcoholic beverages. When asked if they have drunk surgical spirits or meths, the average alcoholic will say 'Thank God, I have never sunk to that yet.'

> London County Council (1964)

These were words that rang fierce bells with us both as we shared, albeit only partially, in the rejection and sense of abandonment of so many. David, however, unlike me, had already experienced a good deal of

rejection through his teenage years with a violent father, followed by periods of homelessness on the streets of East London. These early
experiences, and no doubt other later ones, contributed to his times of
depression, restlessness and intense anger.

In 1964, I met two young heroin addicts, the two sons of my church
warden in Shoreditch. One managed to come off, the other overdosed on
methadone and died. Through them I found that I was quickly getting to
know all the intravenous addicts in East London. Some years later, after a
number had died, a powerful feeling of overwhelming darkness came
over me, a sense, in part, I suppose, of empathy with the slow suicide of
heroin, with the urge to annihilation which was well captured by The
Velvet Underground in their song 'Heroin':

> I have made a decision.
> I am going to try to nullify my life.

In the same period, the folk singer Bert Jansch drew crowds regularly to
Les Cousins Club in Greek Street, Soho, when he sang 'Needle of Death'.
Some of our own feelings were expressed in a pamphlet *Teenagers and
Drugs*, published by the Association of Education Committees in 1966,
the only publication which David and I co-authored.

As a priest, working in the second half of the 1960s, I found that an area
for which my 'training' had not prepared me well was that of ascetical
theology. We had, of course, had lectures on 'spiritualia', but there had
been little attention to the need for a profound inner exploration of one's
own inner depths if one was to be of any real use to people in distress and
turbulence. Much of the stress in pastoral theology was on 'doing', on the
nuts and bolts of the pastoral task. But at the heart of the growing drug
culture, surrounded by many people who had lost hope, by others who
were homeless, suicidal, desperately lost, I realized that the kind of
resources which were needed were not so much skills or expertise as
inner stability, exposure to brokenness, ability to cope with darkness and
the dawning awareness that bewilderment was 'another way of knowing'
(Lane, 1998: 4f).

Of course, I do not wish to convey the impression that everything in
these areas of work is dark and dismal. There were, and are, many shafts
of hope, points of ecstasy, rays of light, moments of fun, times of refreshing. Yet now, after 45 years' working in inner city neighbourhoods, I
realize how central is the symbol of darkness.

It is evident at an obvious level, historically and politically. The East End
in particular is linked historically with images of the dark, from William
Booth's 'darkest England' and Jack London's 'people of the abyss' to
the present day. Much of the time, communities, interest groups, subcul-
tures, even whole populations, are literally 'in the dark' about what the

'principalities and powers' are up to in their schemes of 'regeneration' and 'renewal'. The experience of being on the receiving end of other people's decisions, linked to the facade of 'consultation', is common, if not universal, in inner cities. It is combined with a sense, historically rooted and apparently verified, that there is 'nothing that we can do', and that those in power – the property developers, central government, transnational companies, or the local state with its 'hangers-on' – will get their way. There is a sense of paralysis rather than apathy, the fruit, in many cases, of years of struggle, of banging one's head against a brick wall.

In a letter in *The Times*, published on 9 November 1966, I described our experience at that time:

> Those who daily face the problems of the young drug taker are finding the obstacles almost insurmountable: hours and days spent ringing round hospitals for admissions; refusals, evasions and interminable delays; addicts whose condition deteriorates and parents whose hearts are broken; doctors who refuse to prescribe, and doctors who prescribe with almost criminal irresponsibility; and an overwhelming sense of hopelessness and despair among those who know the drug scene closest.

I ended my letter with these words:

> The situation can be exaggerated and distorted, but it is serious enough ... And perhaps most frightening of all is the fact that many of our best workers in the areas of infection are coming to feel that they are banging their heads against a brick wall. Paralysis, like addiction itself, spreads like a cancer and destroys.

The manifestation of this paralysis in terms of what we have (since the early 1970s) come to call 'spirituality' is brought out in a reflection by the Liverpool Passionist priest Austin Smith, written against the background of the 1981 uprisings there (Smith, 1983). In the midst of the events, Smith reread St John of the Cross's *The Dark Night of the Soul*, and found that it summed up his response to the 'riots'. The inability to see clearly or make definite progress, combined with an intensity of desire, outrage and yearning for justice, is, I think, the political form of today's 'dark night of faith' as it is experienced by many urban (and other) people. The forces which oppress, dehumanize and dominate are powerful and entrenched. Before they can be overcome and transcended, there has to be a corporate and personal *ascesis*, a sharing in darkness and dereliction, in helplessness and emptiness, a real 'famine of the spirit'.

The classic statement of the centrality of the 'dark night of the soul' within the Western Christian tradition is, of course, that of St John of the Cross in the 16th century. For John, the dark night was not a state of psychological disturbance such as deep depression, though it could be, and often is, associated with a range of psychological conditions (Meadows, 1984; Stone, 1998). It is certainly a condition of inner turbulence, upheaval and confusion, characterized by the collapse of familiar ways of praying and feeling, and by the onset of a state of numbness and dereliction. Yet for John, the dark night was an essential part of the life of faith, a sign of progress and of creative, if painful, movement. As earlier forms of spiritual life died, the person moved into a sphere of freedom as the Holy Spirit increasingly took over her heart and life. John was critical of those who tried to push the person back to the earlier religious disciplines and structures, not realizing that they had been transcended and had to be abandoned. His book *The Ascent of Mount Carmel*, of which *The Dark Night of the Soul* is an integral part, is an account of progress, through confusion and upheaval, towards spiritual maturity.

St John of the Cross assumed that his followers and readers were baptized and faithful Christians, seeking holiness and Christian discipleship. In the 21st century, many of his assumptions are called into question in the fragmented state of the religious world and the complexity around spiritual traditions. Many people, within, outside or on the edges of religious traditions are experiencing darkness and spiritual famine but have no disciplines or resources with which to respond to such experiences. Similarly, it probably did not occur to John that, in a post-Christendom period, the experience of the dark night might become corporate, institutionalized, even global, and not just personal. But this seems to be our predicament in the West: a state of uprootedness, of spiritual disintegration, where many exist in spiritual and moral destitution, speaking (in MacIntyre's words) the languages of everywhere and of nowhere (MacIntyre, 1981).

The dark night of the soul is always a painful process, but perhaps much more so in the post-Christian epoch where familiar landmarks and scaffolds have been removed or mislaid. I do not believe that our situation is hopeless, rather that we need to return to older sources of wisdom and insight, and slowly recover and rebuild structures of guidance and nourishment. Because, as MacIntyre has rightly said, there are 'no large remedies' for our predicament: the future must lie with small provisional communities of prayer, discernment, discourse and support (MacIntyre, 1981).

There is, however, another tradition within Christianity involving darkness, without whose influence St John of the Cross might never have written. This is the ancient Eastern tradition of *agnosia*, unknowing, which we find in Dionysius the Areopagite, Gregory of Nyssa and others, and which emerges in the West in the 14th-century tract *The Cloud of Unknowing*. Here darkness is not merely the absence, but the transcendence, of speech. From the kataphatic, that which we can say, about God and the life of the Spirit, we move towards the apophatic, that which cannot be spoken. We move into the silence of the divine darkness.

As in St John, so in the early Eastern orthodox teachers, the darkness is not the opposite of the light but is the way in which infinite light is perceived by finite humanity. In the orthodox tradition, 'God' is always beyond naming – the Cappadocians even debated whether the word 'God' should be abandoned because of the danger of idolatry, of mistaking the name for the reality – and beyond all that can positively be said. Beyond utterance and symbol lies the world of the apophatic, the world of silence and darkness. David Brandon, like many other Western people, was led towards the way of Zen, partly because of his awareness of the inadequacy, brokenness and fragility of language and symbol.

Let me return to my own experience as a priest in the East End, working with homeless people, drug users, people with 'mental health problems' – an experience common to us all, yet experienced most intensely and most painfully by some of us to whom are given such labels as 'psychotic' and 'manic depressive'. The work of priesthood, here as everywhere, is one primarily of presence rather than of skill and function, and at the heart of Christian priesthood is the encounter with darkness, specifically the dying of Christ and his descent into hell, those events which must precede resurrection.

One of the real dangers in any form of ministry, Christian or not, is that of excessive talk, the temptation to verbal domination which besets the 'caring professions'. By our very articulation, itself a form of power, we can seek to overcome and crush inarticulate and voiceless people. In so doing we become one of the 'disabling professions' of which Illich wrote and of which David was so well aware (Brandon, 1976).

We speak glibly and insensitively about sharing another's darkness. We can never do this fully, for no person can ever know fully what is going on in the deep regions of another's being. Yet there is an affinity and solidarity which develops as a by-product of a common experience of darkness, even though the precise forms may differ. In the very process of entering the darkness of the spirit, we come to know and understand better the predicament of those whose darkness is perceived as terrible and as something thrust upon them, something they did not freely choose or desire. Unless this darkness is in some ways shared, no amount of 'training', no acquisition of skills and techniques will help the pastor, priest or carer. All they will do is provide him or her with more resources with which to do more damage to people.

An important aspect of living 'in the dark' is the recognition that we do not have all the answers, that we are not in control of a corpus of knowledge, and that much of the time we are baffled and have nothing of use to say. Hence the importance of what Ignatius of Antioch, the early

Christian writer, called 'a theology of silence'. Darkness and silence are close. Of course, there is no virtue in silence as such. Silence can be unhelpful, cruel, embarrassing and cold. There is a silence that is the bitter fruit of resignation in the face of oppression. Yet there is a silence that grows from humility and gentleness, which recognizes the importance of receiving, listening to and respecting what the other has to say. Over-swift vocal response is usually glib and unhelpful.

In pastoral care, silence is critical. If we are to be genuine carers, we need to slow down and absorb situations, to learn how to be passive and receptive. It is true that the Greek word from which 'passion' and 'passionate' derive means 'suffer', but its root is related to passivity. It is the opposite of active. To be active is to do something; to be passive is to do nothing, to receive. Of course, I realize that without a context these sentences can be dangerous and wrong. There are times when drastic action is called for. There are times to speak loudly, times to 'rage against the dying of the light'. I am not recommending silence and passivity as universal postures. I am myself a lifelong activist and much of my energy still goes into campaigns and struggles for justice. All I am trying to do is correct a distorted emphasis on speech and action, and to stress that silence and receptiveness are important parts of being human, and of being loving instruments of care.

We need to lose our fear of silence, as of darkness and solitude, and this can only come through patient and disciplined practice. I once said at a meeting of my support group, 'I don't think I have got the balance right between the active side of me and the contemplative.' A woman who has known me for a long time commented, 'By introducing the word "balance" you have confused the discussion. It is not a question of balance. What you need to learn is how to integrate, to do the things you do in a more contemplative, reflective way. You may end up doing more, not less, but it will be done in a more reflective way.'

I am sure she was right. One of the most serious dangers confronting those who minister in the city is that their lives come to be built on frenzy and compulsive busy-ness. This usually leads to a lack of focus, a tendency to accumulate more and more things, a collapse of reflection and the cultivation of a personal culture of obligatory tiredness. This personal culture then becomes socially infectious, so that one may communicate little to others other than one's own exhaustion – not a very kind gift to people who may already have enough problems of their own. The practice of silence and solitude, including the cultivation of inner stillness and inner peace, is a vital component of an urban spirituality.

There is a dialectic in pastoral care between speech and silence. The related issue of order and chaos also has to be seen dialectically. In much popular writing and rhetoric, chaos is the enemy. Much work with homeless drug users is described as work with those with 'chaotic lifestyles'. Yet destructive chaos is often the direct result of oppressive order. Much social and political theory has emphasized order at the expense of justice, mercy and truth.

Recent work in quantum physics has stressed the positive value of chaos. The psychologist and theologian Diarmuid O'Murchu (1997), and the community development worker Alison Gilchrist, have applied some of this thinking to personal and social care and to the processes of change in society. Gilchrist's work has important implications for pastoral theology, and provides, albeit not intentionally, a bridge between pure science and pastoral care. Gilchrist sees networking as a way of handling uncertainty and ambiguity, and even defines community as a complex system at the edge of chaos. She argues that community development cannot be realized through business plans or the fulfilment of specific performative criteria, but is about helping disadvantaged populations move towards the 'edge of chaos' by sowing and nurturing dynamic, integrated and socially diverse networks, which are neither utterly confusing nor frozen rigid. It is human horticulture rather than social engineering (Gilchrist, 2000).

It seems to me that 'the edge of chaos' is where we often are, in pastoral care. Yet much of our pastoral work has been shaped within a framework of a culture of order. Metanoia, usually translated as 'repentance' in most English versions of the New Testament, means a complete reversal: transformation, turn-around, revolution. The closest Greek equivalent is paranoia. To be paranoid literally means to be out of your mind; to be 'metanoid' means to be renewed in your mind, transformed, put together again, clothed in one's right mind. But the process is painful and filled with conflict.

A central mark of Christian existence is prayer, which, at its simplest and most profound, means attention to God. I have focused in this essay on themes of darkness, silence, chaos and the inarticulate, and these themes are at the very core of prayer. It is here that we see, in its sharpest form, 'the need to press on in darkness and formlessness in an absence of obvious meaning' (Williams, 1982: 92). While words and symbols, and the combination of both in rite and ceremony in what is called liturgy, are integral elements in prayer, there is an apophatic core which is silent, unspeakable, beyond concept, a point where even symbols are stretched to breaking point.

Out of chaos may come something new and creative. This is one reason why the spiritual guides in the classic tradition insist that there is no easy, calm, 'straight' path to divine union, but only the way of turbulence, upheaval, metanoia. The focus is on attentive waiting on God, in silence. This is not an 'advanced' form of piety reserved for initiates or the very holy: it is the simplest way of praying, to which, from excess of verbal complexity, we need to return.

As a Christian who believes that the word became flesh, and consequently that divine and human are joined, I see a close link between the
attentive listening dimension in prayer and the equivalent in human
intercourse. In both there is a need to cultivate a spirit of attentiveness, a
spirit which takes each person with the utmost seriousness, respect and
reverence.

In writing on Christian ministry at the dawn of the 21st century, I see
two conflicting approaches. One is essentially functionalist, managerial
and bureaucratic – an approach represented by Gordon Kuhrt's *An
Introduction to Christian Ministry* (Kuhrt, 2000). This book, written from
a narrow and insular managerial perspective, has a semi-official status in
the Church of England. The nature of the people of God, and all the
things that matter in ministry, receive little or no attention. Nor is there
any attention to prayer – so central in Michael Ramsey's book *The
Christian Priest Today* (Ramsey, 1972), to which the author refers, and
which has, mercifully, been recently reprinted. Ramsey's book, for many
years the best-known and most valued 'introduction to Christian ministry'
within Anglicanism, is so much deeper, so theologically and spiritually
richer, and so much more exciting than Kuhrt's book that even to
compare the two is an insult to Ramsey's memory. Ramsey's whole understanding of priesthood was steeped in prayer. 'Prayer' does not even
appear in the index of Kuhrt's book, and is dealt with briefly in a section
about 'dangers'. The Eucharist, that sacrament which is at the very heart
of priestly identity, gets little attention. It is striking that, in the cover pictures of ministerial hands in various positions, the conspicuous absentee
is any picture of hands holding bread and wine.

The other approach, more deeply rooted in the approach to mystery,
prayer and 'the holy' is reflected in Bill Countryman's *Living on the Border
of the Holy* (Countryman, 1999). Here, Christian priesthood is located
within the wider context of human priesthood, and the whole thrust of the
work is towards an essentially mystical understanding of the work of the
priest and indeed of religious life itself. Reading Countryman took me back
to my early years as a priest when I read Ulrich Simon's *A Theology of
Auschwitz* (Simon, 1967). I found this book more penetrating, more per-
ceptive, about the nature of priesthood than all the 'how to do it' books.
Simon points to the priest in the concentration camp, stripped of bread
and wine and all the external paraphernalia of priestly work.

> The priestly ideal uses and converts the nothingness which the world of
> Auschwitz offers. Here the priest's sacerdotal dedication encounters the vac-
> uum with self-sacrifice ... The priest at the camp counts because he has no
> desires of self-importance and gives life because he stands already beyond
> extermination. He is the exact opposite to the king-rat. The hour of darkness
> cannot take him by surprise since he has practised silence in darkness.

Between Calvary and Auschwitz lie all the lesser darknesses and deaths – and the hope of resurrection.

References

Brandon D (1976) Zen in the Art of Helping. London: Routledge.

Countryman LW (1999) Living on the Border of the Holy. Harrisburg, PA: Morehouse.

De-la-Noy M (1990) Michael Ramsey: a portrait. London: HarperCollins.

Ecclestone A (1980) The Night Sky of the Lord. London: Darton, Longman and Todd.

Gilchrist A (2000) The well-connected community: networking to the 'edge of chaos'. Unpublished manuscript.

Kuhrt G (2000) An Introduction to Christian Ministry. London: Church House Publishing.

Lane BC (1998) The Solace of Fierce Landscapes: exploring desert and mountain spirituality. Oxford: Oxford University Press.

London County Council (1964) Crude Spirit Drinkers. London: London County Council.

MacIntyre A (1981) After Virtue. Notre Dame, IN: University of Notre Dame Press.

Meadows MJ (1984) The dark side of mysticism: depression and the dark night. Pastoral Psychology 33(Winter): 105–125.

O'Murchu D (1997) Quantum Theology. New York: Crossroad.

Ramsey M (1972) The Christian Priest Today. London: SPCK.

Simon U (1967) A Theology of Auschwitz. London: Gollancz.

Smith ACP (1983) The church and powerlessness. The Way 23(3): 207.

Stone HW (1998) Depression and spiritual desolation. Journal of Pastoral Care 52(4): 389–396.

Williams R (1982) Resurrection. London: Darton, Longman and Todd.

PART THREE
Journeys

And I said to a man who stood at the gate of the year:

'Give me a light that I may tread safely into the unknown.'

And he replied: 'Go out into the darkness and put your hand into the hand of God. That shall be to you better than a light, and safer than a known way.

Minnie Louise Haskins

You think the goal justifies the means, even the vile means. You are wrong: The goal is in the path on which you arrive at it. Every step of today is your life of tomorrow. No great goal can be reached by vile means.

Wilhelm Reich

There is no dichotomy between spirit and flesh, no split between Godhead and the World ... Spiritual union is found in life within nature, passion, sensuality – through being fully human, fully one's self.

Starhawk

CHAPTER 6

Craving

IAN BEECH

Ian Beech teaches psychiatric nursing in the University of Glamorgan in South Wales and also works clinically with people in depression. He hopes that he may, in some small way, help people on their journey of recovery.

Preamble

The story of the Buddha's path to enlightenment is one that has become better known over the past 40 years in the West. The prince Siddartha Gautama's protected, palatial existence is disrupted by what have become known as the four sights: ageing, sickness, death and the renunciate spiritual life. Encountering the four sights convinces the spoiled brat that there is more to life than hedonistic pleasure and persuades him to leave his cosy, sheltered life to follow the path of renunciation to seek the means by which to conquer these horrors. He succeeds in breaking the circle of samsara, wherein people spend their time in suffering from one lifetime to another.

We move forward 2500 years and find that the beleaguered Himalayan country of Tibet is occupied by the Chinese and that thousands of Tibetans have been imprisoned, tortured and killed by the invaders (Tsering Shakya, 1999; Ani Pachen and Donnelley, 2000). Yet the spiritual and temporal leader in exile of the Tibetan people smiles calmly and says that he feels more compassion for the perpetrators of such acts than for the victims (HH the Dalai Lama, 1996).

Common sense appears to tell us, therefore, that there must be something to this Buddhism. Perhaps it can help us to lose our unhappiness, to learn how to put a stop to the craving that characterizes so much of our dissatisfaction with our lives. Meanwhile, as Thomas Szasz has been reminding us for many years, there has, in the West, been a separation of state and religion to the extent that psychiatry has now taken over many of the functions of religion in society (Szasz, 2000). In view of Szasz's assertion, perhaps Buddhism may even provide us with the basis of helping people to live a spiritual life while equipping us to cope with the pressures of modern life in the absence of the influence of the Christian church.

It might be instructive to consider some of the underlying assumptions that back up some of these ideas. It seems that:

- there is a view being held that sees Buddhism as a single religion that can provide a single set of outcomes for Westerners in search of peace of mind;
- there is a belief that Buddhism is good for your mental health;
- Buddhist practitioners from other countries and cultures are imbued with special qualities that shine out as an example to Westerners;
- Buddhism, at the very least, can make mundane lives interesting and so protect us against the vagaries of finding our existence somehow meaningless.

In this chapter, we will, in particular, consider the approach to Buddhism known as Vajrayana Buddhism, which is essentially Tantric Buddhism and Dzogchen, founded predominantly in Tibet, but strands of which exist within certain Japanese approaches to the path (e.g. Shingon). In this we will be considering the assumptions above, and also the guru–disciple relationship and the basic teachings on emptiness and form.

The homogeneity of Buddhism?

In one sense, there is no such thing as Buddhism. Such a concept is a construction of Western society. In countries where the Buddha's teachings have been followed for centuries, people refer to Buddha dharma or simply dharma, which, roughly translated, means the way or teaching of the Buddha (Bercholz and Kohn, 1994). Even if, for the purposes of convention, we use the term 'Buddhism', we find that there are many different approaches to Buddhism. As Rig'dzin Dorje (2001) tells us, the different traditions of Buddhism can be disconcertingly contradictory.

Here, we are concerned primarily with Vajrayana Buddhism, and this can be differentiated from many other forms of Buddhism, for example in Vajrayana we may well encounter a Buddhist who drinks alcohol and eats meat. This in itself can be confusing to people who encounter this form of Buddhism for the first time. Some of the practices involved in Vajrayana can also be confusing, since coupled with silent sitting meditation (shiné) there can also be a lot of noise and the use of a variety of musical instruments, including trumpets made out of human thigh bones. This can create considerable confusion in those who have a preconceived view of Buddhists as a fairly peaceable, meditative lot.

In one sense, all Buddhist teachings are the same. The starting point for this idea is emptiness and form. One of the most well-known sutras (written teachings) in Buddhism is the Heart Sutra, which states:

> Form is emptiness; emptiness is also form. Emptiness is no other than form; form is no other than emptiness. In the same way, feeling, perception, formation and consciousness are emptiness.

Bercholz and Kohn (1994: 155)

In many forms of Buddhism the idea that there is no differentiation between emptiness and form (things and nothingness, happiness and sadness, male and female), i.e. that everything has a non-dual nature, is arrived at in a methodical, analytical way. For example, if students are asked to consider an object such as a cart, then to imagine the wheels being removed from the cart; does the cart still exist? What if the axle is removed? What about the seat, etc.? Through this analytical approach and meditation, practitioners eventually come to realize the non-dual nature of existence and become enlightened. But this may take many lifetimes.

Vajrayana Buddhism takes the view that all humans are beginninglessly enlightened but that we adopt ways of deluding ourselves that we are not. Therefore the Buddhist path for a Vajrayana Buddhist relies on having direct experience of the non-dual state and finding strategies to enable this to happen.

We all have experience of form – it is the solid stuff with which we are surrounded, but it is also the psychological and emotional security blanket with which we surround ourselves. When we encounter anything new, whether it be something solid or an experience, we file it away in our own personal filing cabinet in drawers such as 'stuff I like' and 'stuff I don't like'. As such, we construct our view of how the world is. Emptiness is a little more difficult for us to understand because it is generally outside our everyday experience, and even when we experience it we try desperately to turn it into form. So when we experience form disappearing – for example, the death of someone we like having around, or the disappearance of some of our certainties, such as status, relationship, job, money – we feel unease and discomfort and try to make sense of how things are for us in the world at that moment. In other words, we try to take that experience of emptiness and turn it into form. This is exactly what psychotherapy is attempting to do by trying to make sense (switch into form) of the discomfort (emptiness) we experience in our lives and allow us to move forward into a more effective comfort zone. So enterprises such as psychotherapy are, in effect, antithetical to Vajrayana Buddhism because, in Buddhist terms, they are merely attempting to continue to shore up people's delusions of unenlightenment. But Vajrayana Buddhism teaches that emptiness and form are one and the same; you cannot have one without the other unless you delude yourself. As the Scottish comedian Billy Connolly points out, there is no such thing as bad weather, just useless coats. Good and bad are constructions we have placed on our experiences in an effort to maintain our comfort. There is an old Tibetan proverb that shows us that in spite of all our efforts non-dual reality breaks through:

> A man sat in his house wishing life was better. A knock came on the door and there was a beautiful young woman. He asked who she was and what she wanted. She exclaimed 'I am the good luck lady and I bring good luck, wealth, fame and happiness to whoever gives me a roof over my head.' She came to live with him whereupon his luck changed. Eventually he married her and became rich, healthy and famous and became one of the most well-known and respected men in the area.
>
> He was settling down to a life of ease when one day a knock came on the door and, on opening it, he was confronted by the ugliest, foulest hag he had ever met. She said 'I am searching for somewhere to live, I am the bad luck lady.' He told her to try the next village because he had no room. But she replied 'That's not possible I'm afraid, I have to live with you because you're married to my sister.'

Ngakpa Chögyam (1995)

Is Buddhism good for your mental health?

Buddhism is not a panacea for the mental health distress of the world. Clifford (1984) has demonstrated that within Tibetan medicine, for example, there is a long tradition of explanation and treatment of both mental and physical distress. There would hardly be a necessity for a Tibetan medical approach to psychiatry if Buddhism in itself could somehow inoculate people against mental disease. As we have already seen in Vajrayana, because of its engagement with the interplay between form and emptiness, there may be a good deal of disease.

As David Brandon considered elsewhere in this volume (in a far more erudite way than I can) when someone is attempting to use a spiritual path in some way to promote self-improvement or to make his/herself feel better, this is what Chögyam Trungpa (1991) has called spiritual materialism. Roughly speaking, spiritual materialism can be seen as the adoption of the spiritual path for the end of making the person feel better. But as we have already seen, this is merely a form-based exercise of redefining oneself as a spiritual person. Ngakpa Chögyam and Khandro Dechen (1997) refer to this as adopting an artificial Buddhist personality; in other words, wearing Buddhist regalia such as prayer beads and attempting to hide anger and aggression behind a facade of Buddhist placidness.

Adopting an artificial Buddhist personality generally leads to a person trying to pick and mix his or her spiritual path by trying to find the bits of various traditions that make the person feel good and rejecting the bits of the teaching that might be problematic. In adopting such actions, are not people simply doing with Buddhism what some people do with Christianity when they attend church for an hour on Sunday then ignore their religion until next Sunday? That is, rejecting the inconvenient parts like guilt and loving thy neighbour, and tailoring their spirituality into a meaningless, mushy cotton wool with which to wrap themselves in warmth.

His Holiness the Dalai Lama has put forward the view that all major religions have something to offer individuals and that indeed it might be preferable for a Westerner to follow a Christian spiritual tradition than to engage with Buddhism (HH the Dalai Lama, 1997). His reasons for this are that it is culturally easier for someone to follow the predominant religion than to swim against the tide. In this, he is recognizing that a religious path is a discipline with constraints and barriers and not simply a cosy feelgood zone, and that following a spiritual path is difficult enough when it is culturally embedded and generally more difficult if it is imported from another culture.

The enlightened Easterner

As David Brandon points out in Chapter 2, there is a projected mystique surrounding Tibetan lamas and Japanese Zen masters. There is no 'f' in Tibetan (the language does not possess the sound), and it seems that this describes the reaction of some people when they come to a Buddhist group and find the lama to be a Westerner – 'there's no effin Tibetan!' This is an interesting phenomenon because presumably everyone engaged in the Buddhist path is hoping to achieve enlightenment. At the same time, however, there is a belief held that there is something special about the lama or master from the East, which must surely mitigate against a Westerner achieving enlightenment. Maybe this is simply an indication of it being early days in the spread of Buddhism to the West. Perhaps early

Christians felt cheated unless Galileans gave them teachings. Or perhaps it is an indication of some people's desire to equate Buddhism with the exotic and interesting because of its novelty value. It is a fact, for example, that Buddhist groups who advertise themselves as tantric practitioners regularly attract interest from people who are rather more intrigued by the word tantric than Buddhist.

In Vajrayana Buddhism, as we have seen, the practitioner is attempting to attain the non-dual state of the realization of the indivisibility of emptiness and form. This involves finding ways of experiencing directly the non-dual state, which is uncomfortable for people. How does the person know how to do this and how does the person know what is likely to work? This is where the guru–disciple relationship enters into Buddhism. The guru–disciple relationship is central to Vajrayana. The disciple has to enter into 'pure view' with respect to the guru. This requires the disciple viewing the guru as an enlightened being. The reason for this is so that any request made by the guru of the disciple is not seen as being made out of the personal likes or dislikes of the guru but out of the requirement to mirror the disciple's enlightened state to him or her (Rig'dzin Dorje, 2001). Perhaps this is why Western students find it easier to enter into pure view with Eastern gurus, because they may appear to be somewhat exotic and different and not prone to going about dressed in jeans. It is instructive here to consider the tale of Chögyam Trungpa. When he arrived in the UK and set up the Samye Ling Centre he was viewed as a Trulku (reincarnation of an enlightened being) and as the most able of all the Tibetan lamas to transmit Buddhist teachings to the West. Trungpa then proceeded to stop wearing monastic robes, to take a wife and to be seen drinking alcohol. This caused great consternation in Buddhist circles (Snelling, 1987). It appears that the guru was exposed as having feet of clay. However, from the perspective of Vajrayana, his behaviour was not that of someone losing the spiritual path, but rather of a guru who was providing for his disciples the direct experience of the non-dual state. But because of the discomfort of the disciples this had to be conceived of by them as being un-lama-like behaviour. Indeed, Rig'dzin Dorje (2001) states that it is not the quality of the lama that is essential but the ability of the student to enter pure view. So it is possible for the guru to be a complete charlatan, but if the student can maintain pure view enlightenment is possible.

The story of Chögyam Trungpa, however, cuts to the very core of the paradox of Buddhism for many people taking the decision to follow the Buddhist path. People take the path with the desire to lose their suffering, and see it as a means by which to lose that suffering. However, the very desire to lose suffering is, according to Buddhist teachings, a cause for suffering. Therefore when the path itself becomes uncomfortable they find themselves in conflict with the teaching of the guru, yet that discomfort has to be experienced in order to enter the non-dual state.

Meaningful (non) existence

The ultimate expression of non-duality is the experience of no self. One of our surest form-based conceptions is of our own existence. Indeed, in Western society the existence of self is the one thing of which, since Descartes, we have been certain (Rolfe, 2000). Yet in Buddhism the solidity of self in terms of form is untenable. Practitioners in Vajrayana will be encouraged to meditate on impermanence of self by the guru. For example, a practitioner may be asked to collect a series of photographs of him or herself from infancy to present day. Starting with a baby photograph, the practitioner is asked to meditate on how much of the baby in the picture is present in the practitioner today. Moving forward through the toddler phase, the first school photograph, etc., the practitioner is asked to consider at what point it can be said that the practitioner is the same person as in any of the photographs. The practitioner comes to the realization that everything is impermanence, that each moment is death and rebirth and that there is no constant sense of self.

A sense of no self can be extremely liberating in many ways. For example, it allows the practitioner to lose the need to portray him- or herself as some consistent entity in the face of situations and to become freely reacting to situations. However, for a person who is suffering from mental distress, the concept of no self can be extremely problematic. Mental distress, whether it takes the form of low mood or hearing voices or having beliefs that differ from those around the person, shares a common factor, which is a sense and awareness of self. Depression, for example, is a state wherein the person self-monitors constantly. 'How do I feel?', 'Am I worse than yesterday?' and 'I have no future and this is a threat to me' are all common feelings found in people described as being in depression. In *The Seduction of Madness*, Podvoll (1990) uses examples of people in an outpatient department who would no doubt attract a variety of psychiatric diagnoses ranging from mania to schizophrenia. In each description of the people concerned, the strength of the sense of self shines through, even if the self is seen as misguided or deluded. If people are approaching Buddhist practice out of a desire to gain control of themselves or their lives by the use of techniques that might seem to promote self-control such as meditation, then they are likely to find that life is not controllable, and that, as Ngakpa Chögyam (1988: 3) states:

> Shi-né (Tibetan Buddhist meditation) is our treatment for our addiction to thought patterns.

But since people are fixated with their thoughts and self-monitoring, going without these can be experienced as intensely boring or frustrating.

One of the things that Buddhist meditation techniques teach is to allow thoughts to appear and disappear without following them, and to simply sit and be. Some people may find the process relaxing and this in itself may be therapeutic to someone who is anxious by nature, but surely no more so than the various relaxation techniques available within the realms of psychotherapy, psychiatry and nursing.

The combination of no-self and the guru–disciple relationship is a heady brew. If the teachings are approached from the perspective of someone entrenched in needing rescue from a series of problems in life, pure view will be impossible and the person will require of the guru that solutions be produced for those problems. At some point the guru will provide an unacceptable challenge to the student's reference points and the relationship will break down or the student will become mired in distress. A distorted sense of self in the guru–disciple relationship results in resentment of the guru as some kind of misleading Svengali figure. This is because we live with a myth that we have freedom of choice, and any commitment to one particular path must, of necessity, reduce freedom rather than facilitate freedom (Rig'dzin Dorje, 2001). In fact, freedom of choice does not allow for total freedom, because every time we make a choice in life we cut off options as well as open them up. If we choose to stay in bed, we miss the TV programme, bus, front of the queue at the sales.

Indeed, to be ready to take on the Vajrayana path the person must be successful at samsara. This means rather than being mired in suffering, the person must have experienced happiness, sadness, indeed the full range of human emotions, and then to have found how impossible it is to stabilize happiness. Having attempted to do this we find how difficult it is and how undesirable it ultimately becomes. As the old Chinese proverb states, 'Be careful what you wish for, you might just get it.'

Finding refuge

A person suffering from mental distress is in effect attempting to seek refuge from that distress. It is tempting to seek refuge from that distress in Buddhism, with its seeming calm and gentle approach to the alleviation of suffering. There is, however, no more sense in finding refuge from mental distress in Buddhism than in Christianity. Teachings on personal responsibility, forgiveness of others and ultimate redemption from personal sin contain many aspects that may be helpful to some people in alleviating their distress. However, to use a spiritual path for an end is missing the point of a spiritual path, for it is a path not an aim. Rig'dzin

Dorje (2001), for example, has suggested that it might be appropriate for someone thinking of engaging with Vajrayana to engage in some form of psychotherapy as a preparation for the path. It is tempting, however, for someone to seek refuge in psychotherapy in the same way that a person might seek refuge in Buddhism. You can take refuge in either but not both.

There may be useful techniques available to people in distress that can be taken from Buddhism as from Christianity, Judaism, Islam, etc. But the important point is that these are techniques that are age-old pieces of wisdom, which may help a person to deal with immediate problems. But a spiritual path is a journey without goal (Chögyam Trungpa, 1981); it may make the person feel better but that would not be the aim, and to start on the journey with that as the aim would be a recipe for disappointment. As Ngakpa Chögyam and Khandro Dechen (1999) say, you have to take full responsibility when you approach Vajrayana Buddhism. You wouldn't join the marines and then cry that you didn't expect people to shoot at you. You might, on the other hand, take the physical training from marine basic training and use it to make yourself feel fitter. That wouldn't make you a marine.

References

Ani Pachen and Donnelley A (2000) Sorrow Mountain. St Helens: Doubleday.

Bercholz S and Sherab Chödzin Kohn (1994) Entering the Stream: an introduction to the Buddha and his teachings. London: Rider.

Chögyam Trungpa (1981) Journey Without Goal: the tantric wisdom of the Buddha. Boston, MA: Shambhala.

Chögyam Trungpa (1991) Crazy Wisdom. Boston, MA: Shambhala.

Clifford T (1984) Tibetan Buddhist Medicine and Psychiatry: the diamond healing. York Beach: Weiser.

HH the Dalai Lama (1996) Beyond Dogma: the challenge of the modern world. London: Souvenir Press.

HH the Dalai Lama (1997) The Four Noble Truths. London: Thorsons.

Ngakpa Chögyam (1988) Journey into Vastness: a handbook of Tibetan meditation techniques. Shaftsbury: Element.

Ngakpa Chögyam (1995) Wearing the Body of Visions. New York: Aro Books.

Ngakpa Chögyam and Khandro Dechen (1997) Spectrum of Ecstasy. New York: Aro Books.

Ngakpa Chögyam and Khandro Dechen (1999) Even a whole chicken might not be enough for the servant of the sun. Vision: Magazine Of The Non-Monastic Traditions Of Buddhism, Summer: 5–14.

Podvoll E (1990) The Seduction of Madness. New York: HarperCollins.

Rig'dzin Dorje (2001) Dangerous Friend: the teacher–student relationship in Vajrayana Buddhism. Boston, MA: Shambhala.

Rolfe G (2000) Research, Truth and Authority: postmodern perspectives on nursing. Basingstoke: Macmillan.

Snelling J (1987) The Buddhist Handbook. London: Rider.

Szasz, T (2000) The case against psychiatric power. In Barker P and Stevenson C (eds), The Construction of Power and Authority in Psychiatry. pp. 43–55. Oxford: Butterworth-Heinemann.

Tsering Shakya (1999) The Dragon in the Land of Snows: a history of modern Tibet since 1947. London: Pimlico.

CHAPTER 7

Confession

LIAM CLARKE

Liam Clarke was born in County Louth, Southern Ireland. He was brought up in the Roman Catholic faith prior to the Second Vatican Council in the 1960s, which meant that:

> I was exposed to a range of religious mechanisms calculated to inculcate guilt and instil obedience. It worked for a while. Since early adulthood I have lived and worked in England, slowly growing in appreciation of the depressing consequences that loss of deference to a moral order brings. Distrustful of the postmodernist impulse, yet suspicious of systems purporting to have 'the answers', things become less definite yet more urgent as one proceeds. Contributing to the community of this book has been a challenge, as it has helped me enjoin the past to the present.

Confessing the soul or the psyche?

When I was a small boy in Catholic Ireland in the 1950s, going to confession on a Saturday afternoon was a mixed blessing. There was the satisfying advantage of having one's sins forgiven – the slate wiped clean for another month. The downside, though, was having to voice one's sins to a priest in the fervent hope that he would quickly move over them, prescribe a penance and not ask awkward questions. Often, a group of us – boys of course – would meet outside the church to tentatively inquire of one another exactly what we needed to tell. Was it necessary to mention *certain things* more than others? Despairingly, we concluded that everything needed to be told; there could be no evasion. I think we needed the comfort of these miserable meetings, the shared security in knowing we had all transgressed in most secret and reprehensible ways.

What the good priests made of it all is hard to say, but they seemed to take us in their stride. They differed in their responses of course and I (vaguely) recall a couple of occasions when things didn't go smoothly. One's sins usually invited little priestly comment, except for those that we had nervously discussed outside the church doors. Awkwardly, the odd priest would try and elicit the minute details of these sins and on such occasions one felt only gratitude for the anonymity of the confessional space. These inquisitions nevertheless were sobering experiences and to be avoided at all costs. Such avoidance often led to a degree of motivated forgetting, whereby more risqué sins were only recalled having left the confessional! This, I believed, was not wrong since they had not been *deliberately* forgotten: to my mind, forgetting something meant that you had not thought of it in the first place and this was hardly a fault. Equally, even at this tender (pre-teen) age, I had become a past master at rationalizing sins away, convincing myself that some sins were not *that* bad and, anyhow, hadn't I confessed the very same sins the month before? What was to be gained by repeating myself? More duplicitous was the commitment given towards the end – 'I firmly resolve to offend no more' – knowing that come hell or high water one *would* re-offend. Aware that bodily desires would overrule strength of will, one retreated into self-deception and promised the unpromisable. Caught up in the effects of his murderous act, Shakespeare's Claudius in *Hamlet*, cries out:

> My words fly up, my thoughts remain below:
> Words without thoughts never to heaven go.
>
> Shakespeare (1994: III, iii, l.97)

Psychological evasion was well known to the medieval fathers, who, in the formative period of private confession, invented rules for its governance. Tentler (1977: 88) quotes one such piece of advice:

> After he has heard the confession, let him begin to inquire distinctly and methodically. Nevertheless, I advise that in his questions he not descend to special circumstances and special sins; for many fall severely after such an interrogation who otherwise never would have dreamt of it.

Detailed inquiry into carnal sins was specially cautioned against, with most writers calling on priests to show sympathy and understanding, to be well informed and to seek help when necessary from more learned counsel. Of course the priests differed in terms of their own religious background and:

> Local priests knew that a visiting mission from the Redemptorists or Passionists was different from one preached by Vincentians or Jesuits. The

parishioners knew likewise that one's reception in the confession box would vary with the confessor's stable.

O'Loughlin (2000: 21–22)

One therefore cut one's penitential cloth accordingly.

Such was the ritual of confessing one's sins to a (hopefully) silent stranger in a dark, claustrophobic space – whose clever construction would become apparent years later when I entered psychoanalysis – and, whatever the terrors this space held, it did its job well. Guilt was assiduously inculcated in us: the erotic smell of particular sins acquiring special status. If you ask why we bothered going, why we didn't just hide and pretend that we had, the answer is that we could not: we *had* to go because, if nothing else, absolution provided relief. Indeed, the yearning to confess can often exist, strangely, in its own right: in *Crime and Punishment*, Raskolnikov's urge to confess is instantaneous upon the commission of his crime:

> A strange thought suddenly occurred to him, to get up at once, go to the superintendent, tell him about what had happened last night, and then take him back to his room and show him all the things in the hole in the corner. His impulse was so strong that he even got up to carry it out.

Dostoyevsky (1951: 122–123)

Throughout this novel, confession is pinned to redemption, to rebirth – Lazarus-like rising from states of moral death – through penance and forgiveness. Magarshack recollects a (deleted) passage from Dostoyevsky:

> A criminal as a rule never possesses much willpower, nor can he be said to be always in his right mind. That is why the shameful thought in his mind is so quickly converted into a wicked deed. But no sooner has the crime been committed than repentance begins to gnaw at his heart like a serpent, and the man will die not because of the crime he has committed, but because he has destroyed what is best in him and what still entitles him to be called a human being.

Magarshack (1951: 11)

For us, avoiding confession would hardly have resulted in a loss of human status but it would still have involved, vaguely, some rejection of our spiritual and human upbringing.

Different ways

This is an account of that confession of which I am familiar but which may be less familiar to you. It is an account grounded in the repetitive (monthly) telling of one's sins to a priest in an enclosed box, coupled with the acceptance of whatever penance was meted out. Unfamiliar or not, I think that this form of confessing holds out a fascination grounded as it is in a subterranean world of sin, secrecy, lies and retribution. I emphasize confession and its history from the standpoint of Christian (and especially Roman Catholic) tradition not because I attribute superior status to these, but because I am familiar with them.

I suppose that confession gained its heavy emphasis in Catholic theology partly because its most powerful scriptural source is also that upon which papal authority rests – in Matthew 16: 19, Christ says to Peter: 'And I will give thee the keys of the kingdom; and whatever thou shall bind on earth shall be bound in heaven, and whatever thou shall loose on earth shall be loosed in heaven'. It could be argued – it has for centuries! – that there is much in this that is merely implicit. Nevertheless, within this tradition people have divulged transgressions as part of a church rite for well on 2000 years. Although most explicit in its requirements within the Roman Catholic tradition, confession has featured in other Christian and some non-Christian religions and does, in fact, predate the Christian period considerably.

The ancient world

Discussing the ancient religions (of Egypt), John Noss (1974) refers to the Kingdom of Osiris (about 1025 BC), where judgement is given before the soul gains entry to the 'enchanted fields'. Interestingly, the soul is examined *after* death in the presence of Osiris and concerning issues of goodness and wickedness. The soul declares what is sometimes mistakenly called a 'negative confession': that is, an account of evils which have *not* been committed rather than those that have. After confession the soul is judged and allowed to move on.

Within Jewish tradition, judgement begins on Rosh Hashanah, the day that celebrates the world's creation. O'Dea et al. describe it thus:

> On the most solemn day of the year, the Day of Atonement, which is given over completely to prayer and fasting, the judgement is concluded. From Rosh Hashanah through to Yom Kippur the Jew has repented and sought mercy. He has confessed his sins innumerable times, and has laid himself open before the righteous judge. After a full day of prayer, the worshipper, humbly trusting in God's mercy and goodness, finally bursts out in joyous affirmation: 'The Lord is God, the God of Love, He alone is God'.

O'Dea et al. (1972: 124)

In some religions, atonement is conspicuously absent. For instance:

> Confucianism [does] not provide for private worship or prayer, nor for rites of atonement, confession or self mortification to take away sins.

Graham (1971: 365)

In Confucianism, the moral code is secular, not religious, so that although the flesh is regarded as sinful, something like exposing one's body could lead to shame, but in terms of having violated a social – not religious – code. Similarly, in Buddhism, confession as an outward declaration of sinning is elusive, and preoccupation with the physical world (compared with Christianity) becomes insignificant. After the time of the Buddha himself, essential rules were developed so as to govern the Buddhist priestly order. The wearing of the yellow habit, the shaven head, carrying a begging bowl, daily meditation and the initiate monk's declarative confession: 'I take refuge in the Buddha, I take refuge in the Dhama (the Law of Truth), I take refuge in the Sangha (the Order)' (Noss 1974: 126).

For the Christian tradition, too, there are different (sometimes important) emphases. Comparing the Eastern and Western Churches, Zernov (1971) comments that in the Roman Church the role of the confessor is that of judge. The priest is empowered to absolve penitents and he assigns them a penance in reparation for sins committed. In the Eastern Church (aligned with Rome), the priest is not a judge; he is a witness to the penitent's confession, a fellow Church member whose brotherly advice facilitates repentance.

Within Protestantism, there is no tradition of confession: this reflects the theological emphasis on sinners having direct access to their maker without ministerial intercession. Most of the Protestant reformers accepted only Baptism and the Eucharist as having been instituted by Christ himself. With the exception of the Lutherans, priestly confession was abandoned. Mindful of his desperate struggles to find a right relationship with God, Luther kept faith with confession as an aid to repentance and salvation – he continued to make his confession for the rest of his life – and confession continues to have a role in Lutheran practice.

The Protestant reformers were not so much bothered by the practical abuses of confession, but more its capacity to torment rather than console. Luther condemned the 'gallows sorrow' of traditional confession wherein penitents confess through fear. Sinners should confess, said Luther, because they want to. Luther also condemned confession as an obligatory event. The Pope had commanded (in 1215) at least yearly confession, and to this day Catholics are encouraged to confess frequently. Luther saw obligatory confession as an exercise in power and insisted that people should never feel compelled to confess. His most damaging

perception, however, concerned the futility of engaging in detailed examination of conscience prior to confessing lists of sins most of which were
probably inevitable and over which people had limited control – sins of
lust for example. What joy that would have brought to the psychological
torment of us Catholic adolescents as we strove – over 400 years later – to
profess contrition in the knowledge that we would do *it* again.

What Protestantism urged instead was a general statement of sinfulness
as a prelude (and commitment) to transforming one's life. For the reformers, a hypocritical element suffused the Catholic predilection for regular
confession and they wanted to be done with this. For them, the idea that
a good confession entailed a rigorous examination of conscience and
working up sufficient sorrow was far too anthropocentric. They opted
instead for a passive contrition while accepting the uselessness of this in
the face of God's power. All that could be hoped for was that forgiveness
would be given because of the sinner's belief that it would be: 'justification by faith alone'. This is, I suppose, more consoling than the medieval
tradition and this was what the reformers intended. Yet there are psychological difficulties in displacing responsibility to God: sin breeds guilt –
else why confess? – but guilt is not easy to come by in respect of enjoyable
sins, as Claudius tells us. If encountering a priest is more rather than less
likely to induce shame, might this not work for guilt as well? Might guilt
be psychologically more realized in the presence of another, rather than
standing before God with, so to speak, only the void in between.

Of course, as Catholic schoolboys we too were told: 'The priest does
not forgive sins, God forgives sins'. We never thought to ask the obvious
which was: 'If God forgives sins then why do we need the priest?' We need
him, according to St Thomas Aquinas, because contrition alone does not
produce forgiveness: absolution is a sacrament and a sacrament is a rite;
Jesus *presided* at events and awarded some of his followers special powers enabling them to do likewise. Sacramental confession would be
practised by those specially blessed and this special status would be stip-
ulated as originating in the time of Jesus. Human intermediaries also had
the effect of providing psychological assurance that forgiveness had actually taken place. Having, in my case, been brought up to believe that 'the
priest cannot lie', in addition to the sense of otherness which the priest
bore, there was also an immediacy, an undeniable realness to his pro-
nouncement: 'Ego te absolve'.

The heart of confession

From the beginnings of institutionalized confession, four elements have
been present: first sinners have had to show contrition, second they must

make some form of explicit confession, third they must do penance, fourth the process must be mediated by a priest who pronounces absolution. From the earliest periods of Judeo-Christianity a priest has been regarded as an essential intermediary between the confessant and God.

Commentators typically denote the evolution of confession in three phases: from the first to sixth centuries it is a communal (priest-led) undertaking, then from the seventh to 15th centuries it gradually emerges as a private and repeatable event, with the period from the 16th century to the present reinforcing already time-honoured traditions.

In the early Church, confession was only invoked for very serious transgressions – for example apostasy. The penance usually involved exclusion from the community of the faithful or other serious public penance. Reconciliation with the faithful was allowed (but once only) and on a restricted basis: the reformed individual could not become a clergyman, for example, nor could he contract a marriage or join the military. As Perrin observes:

> The sacramental practice focussed less on the role and the sins of the individual and more on the injury done to, and thus the necessary reconciliation to be had with, the community.
>
> Perrin (1998: 101)

From the start, forgiveness was linked to penance, and not always in that order. In the early and middle periods of Church history, penitential acts were often required *before* forgiveness could be contemplated. And this is not penance as we know it: in his examination of the *Roman Penitential* – one of several manuals (for priests) which categorized sins and suggested appropriate punishments – Tentler (1977: 11) notes the severity and length of particular penances. A cleric guilty of homicide 'shall do penance for ten years, three of these are bread and water'; the layman, for the same crime, gets seven years with three on bread and water. For adultery resulting in childbirth, a cleric gets seven years of penance; without childbirth it is three with one on bread and water. Typical requirements of these lengthy penances were fasting, worship and charitable works. Only on completion could the sinner be given another chance and gain readmittance to the fold; so that at this time a central feature was the regard for sins as serious, even monumental, transgressions and not at all similar to our concept of reeling off lists of venial sins in anticipation of a few short prayers as penance.

Deathbed confessions

Something that characterizes all ages is how confession acts as a psychological comfort: this is seen in the (early) willingness to allow confession for people near death, when little penance is possible. Unsurprisingly, putting off reconciliation until near death became commonplace from the medieval period, perhaps with an eye to avoiding the severe penances. Tentler (1977) states that deathbed confessions imply that confession was not just about defining relationships between the individual and his church but that 'some kind of divine as well as ecclesiastic forgiveness' was also involved. In addition, deathbed confessions 'led to an increased privatisation of the practice of reconciliation in general' (Perrin, 1998: 102). Excluding the wider community necessarily brings with it an emphasis on individuals and a corresponding lessening of concern about communal issues. In this also, we see the roots of confession not only as a means of ridding sins but also, in a very primitive sense, as a means of psychological reassurance. But because of this, deathbed confessions became controversial. St Augustine opposed them, taking the view that there is not much point in giving up sinning if one is no longer in a position to sin and, of course, deathbed penances had (understandably) to be lenient.

Other influences on the development of private confessions came from Ireland, where Christian groups had acquired formal structures less with a bishop at their centre and more in the form of monastic settlements with a strong missionary flavour. O'Dea et al. state that:

> Irish missionaries of the sixth and seventh century introduced the practice [of private confession] to the laity as a whole, and with it a penitential literature which had flourished in Ireland. The practice replaced an earlier public confession of the community and became throughout the middle ages a long training school in introspection and self examination without which Martin Luther and his profound interior religious problems in the sixteenth century would hardly have been possible.
>
> O'Dea et al. (1972: 66)

The medieval period

By the 12th century confession was fairly established as a frequent, private, affair and penitential fasting and lengthy vigils were giving way to shorter penances consisting of prayers. The reasons for this are varied: a more sophisticated theological debate challenged the severity of penances but, equally, the sly observation that lesser penances recruited more confessants may also have prevailed. This falling off in harsher penances led, in turn, to problems of working out how one knew that one had been forgiven: if part of the function of harsh penances was to assuage guilt and diminish anxiety, then the more harsh the penances the more might people feel that their dues had been paid, that the purgatorial tariff had been reduced. As medieval time passed, a state of contrition was starting to be seen as sufficient penance and theologians began to ask – as Luther more forthrightly would later – whether acknowledging sins through a good act of contrition was sufficient grounds for a harmonious relationship between man and God: in effect, was an intermediary ecclesia necessary?

Yet confessing to a priest had existed for centuries and medieval theologians also began the process of finding biblical justification for it. This proved difficult and, perhaps in compensation, the notion of shame was introduced to justify the priestly presence: if telling one's transgressions to a priest induced embarrassment and shame then this might act to exculpate sin. Although it would be debated at length, bishops persistently defended priestly confession in large part to maintain church discipline and control over penitents. At the Fourth Lateran Council in 1215, confession was declared a sacrament and yearly confession to a priest was made mandatory, thus legitimizing confession as an ecclesiastic procedure. Later, the Council of Trent (1545-1563) emphasized the judicial role of the priest and this was heightened by 17th-century declarations by the Holy See that:

> classified any transgression on matters of sexuality as an objectively serious matter constituting mortal sin.
>
> Rausch (1998: 407)

The box

The history of confession until the late middle ages, therefore, is a development from public to private, from occasional to frequent, and from community through to priestly mediation. A stunning innovation, in the 16th century, is the introduction of the confession box. It was largely the creation of Cardinal Borromeo, Archbishop of Milan (1564–1584), working through the Counter-Reformation's Council of Trent. In Borromeo's confessional:

> the person who comes to confess is unseen, unknown

and there is created:

> a visual sense of the judicial nature of confession

where:

> the seated confessor assumed the place of the tribunal: he sat to weight and assess, though still, in theory, to give spiritual comfort.
>
> Tambling (1990: 68)

There is brought about an unequal division of power, for although the confessant is anonymous, he is known by definition as a sinner, as someone seeking forgiveness for sins from someone empowered to give it, even if in another's name. What the confession box allowed was a significant extension of privacy as well as the formalization of elements carried over from the past, for example seating arrangements which prevented priests from looking into the faces of (especially female) penitents. In fact, foreshadowing the confession box was the practice (in some quarters) of trying to ensure that confessor and confessant might not see each other at all. To which we can add the myriad technical debates which now ensued, such as: Were gifts (to priests) to be allowed. Should penitents kneel or was internal submission enough? Should feelings be expressed (priestly amazement, contempt, derision). Should women cover their heads? And so on.

Of greater significance is that an extraordinary space has emerged wherein people's private thoughts find freer expression. As I have suggested, the overlap with classical psychoanalysis is telling: the close proximity of patient to analyst, the social obscurity of both to each other, the frequency of 'sessions', the enclosed space, an air of expectation and even of sanctity. The examination of conscience mirrors the psychoanalytic 'golden rule' of revealing one's secrets and lies, leaving no stone unturned. Of course the crucial difference between confession and therapy is forgiveness: confessants seek absolution, whereas patients seek enlightenment. That said, a successfully resolved transference, in psychoanalytic terms, represents an exculpation of sorts, and the telling of sins is hardly devoid of psychological implications. But what really differentiates the two is that confession affirms man's known place (both spiritually and materially) in the cosmos, whereas psychoanalysis assumes that man's nature to be material and knowable exclusively through human discourse.

Discourse and the 'self'

Until the Enlightenment, the notion of a 'self' – in the way that we conceptualize this today – was unknown. One did not choose a course in life so much as this was preordained through the word of God and its clerical interpretations. When life was 'poor, nasty, brutish and short' (Hobbes, 1651: chapter 13) and no society existed, to speak of, it paid to put one's destiny in the hands of providence. One's 'self', such as it was, counted little, and evil people were seen as possessed by devils or the butt of other unworldly forces. Although private confession had its roots in medieval and earlier periods, it is not surprising that at a time when personal wilfulness played so small a part, private confession was infrequent, and it is only in a post-Cartesian context that confession as individual narrative comes into its own. In the view of John Paul II (1994: 51), Descartes 'marks the beginning of a new era in European thought ... because [he] inaugurated the great anthropocentric shift in philosophy'. Specifically, Rose (1989: 218–220), drawing from Nelson (1965), identifies the emergence of Catholic confession in the middle ages as a major influence on Western modernity, with a growing awareness of man's central place in the wider scheme of things, not divorced from his community but interpreting it from the vantage point of a newfound selfhood. Confessional practice helped create and sustain this notion of the private individual 'measured by deep interiority and feelings' (Tambling, 1990: 2). Rehearsing one's sins – as one was compelled to do – became a device for authoring the self: central to this is Foucault's (1999) assertion that confession is the means by which we subjectify ourselves within power structures. This movement gathered more momentum through the Protestant retrieval of individual (unmediated) conscience, as well as the development of other forms of confession such as writing. Narrating one's misgivings to others, however, may prove difficult where misunderstandings arise concerning terminology or where discrepancies occur between internal versus external attributions of meanings to events and experiences.

Wittgenstein's fideism

While writing the *Philosophical Investigations* (1953), Wittgenstein endeavoured to make a confession of sorts. The confession was to be made to a close circle of friends and family and would involve the telling of a number of venial 'sins' as well as a smaller number of major 'sins', such as his attempts to cover up his Jewish ancestry. Wittgenstein believed in philosophy less as the production of detached treatises and more as something that worked its way through everyday parlance. However, in the world of word games which he proposed, there occur issues of terminological confusion, of working out if a 'true' confession is possible. Believing the Cartesian notion of self to be redundant, Wittgenstein said that what sustained this mistake were endless incursions into language games. Peters observes that providing coherent accounts of ourselves (for example in autobiography):

> fuels omissions, rationalisations, invention: suppressions of salient, raw, stubborn memories which confound the imperial attitude of pretended wholeness or single mindedness.
>
> Peters (1998: 7)

Much of this stems from earlier (for example Kantian) sources: seeing that which we 'wish' to see, remembering the past selectively, and so on. What is added is the 'impossibility' of resolving problems given their inherent instability in language. Language games – occurrences where shared meanings between groups gives language its meaning through usage – are the mechanism by which instabilities and obscurities are clarified: such games (or systems) are impermeable to other systems and their internal truths are not dependent on, or subject to, other systems. O'Grady observes that this has resulted in:

> philosophers of religion, influenced mainly by postmodernism, [arguing] for extreme cognitive diversity from what they regard as the collapse of modernist attempts to establish a universal account of human rationality.
>
> O'Grady (2002: 136)

In this instance, religious belief is no less an act of faith than belief in the explanatory power of science or history: none has any edge over the other. Each exists and is validated within defined areas of human discourse. Emphasizing language difficulties in working through philosophical issues, Wittgenstein denotes admissions of weakness (confession) as a way out. Peters (1998: 7) quotes Wittgenstein thus:

> Anyone in such torment who has the gift of opening his heart, rather than contracting it, accepts the means of salvation in his heart.

However, heart and soul are not synonymous and what seems afoot here is an artistic desire to publicize philosophy as not up to explaining life's mysteries. Within religious frameworks there runs the belief, going back through Luther and St Augustine, that God knows *all* – all the evasions, word games, fabrications – and that what matters is the attempt to confess honestly in the 'knowledge' (the kind that comes through faith) that God hears all. As a child, standing apprehensively with one's friends outside the church, one was in equal parts terrified that God knew that one was about to evade the issue, but that he would forgive us because we were merely human. That said, lingering, hypocritical qualms always followed up on such speculations.

Confession as control

If Wittgenstein's confession was a secular substitution for a religious instinct which eluded him, subsequent philosophy cast religion in even more worldly terms. Foucault begins by (inaccurately) identifying the origins of confession within Catholicism, before proceeding to interpret sacramental rites as mechanisms of control. Unsurprisingly, he describes the examination of conscience as a means by which (Church) oppression is internalized; the process he described goes something like this. In the confession box, violations of the moral order are verbally articulated: the construction of the confessional defines behaviour – especially sexual behaviour – as sinful and prohibited. Words are exchanged in hushed tones (someone outside the box might hear!) and are absorbed and purified through the grace of absolution. The confessant recognizes his sinful nature – so as to report it to the priest – and the exchange indeed consolidates the Church's power over his interior self.

However, we also see a validation of the individual's participation in the Church. The confession box especially represented, on its inventor Borromeo's part, the brilliant psychological insight that intimate contact between the laity and clergy would not only promote disclosure but also enhance the level of the laity's religious standing. Foucault distrusted benevolence, seeing it in Freudian blinkers as a socially connived front, masking propensities for control and coercion. But we must not suppose that people necessarily resent control; they may, in fact, accept it and use it as a cushion against which to test themselves in different ways. Not inconsiderable measures of comfort derive from control where the control is perceived as benevolent. God is all powerful, yes: but God is good.

Confession as therapy

On 23 March 1998 the Associated Press reported Pope John Paul II as saying that confession must not be equated with psychoanalysis or psychotherapy. Declaring that confessors were neither healers nor physicians, the Pope advised priests to direct people in need of such help to competent professionals. What His Holiness was reacting to was the tendency from the 1960s – beginning within liberal Protestantism – to hold organized religion responsible for people's emotional stresses, particularly in respect of human sexuality. Responsible, that is, in the sense of inducing guilt and distress but also bearing a responsibility to respond to distress in an uncritical way. Pastoral care, for some priests, began to take on a less-than-complete religious hue. In particular, the writings of Carl Rogers (1951) became influential, in some cases replacing or at least supplementing conventional manuals of penitential theology. Acceptance (of feelings) within pastoral care relationships became the norm, and with a corresponding falling off of judgementalism (of sins). Pless (2001), a Lutheran pastor, comments that 'the practice of private confession and absolution is regarded by many as an archaic relic left behind by the

Reformation and replaced by more relevant and psychologically sound methods of pastoral care'.

It would be absurd if contemporary religion ignored psychology, and, in fact, the psychology of religion has become an important field of study. In particular, the concept of 'the unconscious' provided 'penitential theologians' with much to think about in respect of the veracity of human confessing. Criminologists, for instance, tell us that some people 'confess' things they haven't done, and the desire (especially on the part of the young) to please or, at least, not displease the priest (father) possesses much psychological significance.

Freud and Jung

Together with Carl Rogers (and antedating him), Freud and Jung are the transformation ground between psychology and religion. In the case of Freud, God is an illusion; in the case of Jung, He/She is a myth. Freud puts great – though not exclusive – emphasis on the sexual instinct, insisting that neurotic dysfunction results from repressing sexual urges. Freud was aware that people varied in how this might affect them; yet, however one sees this, it seems clear that Catholic strictures on sexuality – certainly in the past – induced considerable conflict in young boys and girls. Whereas Freud saw the Super Ego as an impediment, the Church saw it as a happy hunting ground: it recognized that 'conscience doth make cowards of us all', inhibiting and chastising from within and thus mandating good behaviour. Freud, too, saw the point that guilt might obtain civilization but was aware of the repressive price to be paid.

Jung's belief in religion as myth is not always appreciated and he is generally seen as friendly towards Christianity when, in fact, he was really about constructing a cosmology of his own. He taught that man had 'a natural religious function' and that this required expression as much as any of his instincts (Fordham, 1953). He posited a collective unconscious where archetypes (or shadows) operated to influence human behaviour: we could never know this unconscious, but it was unknowing that gave it its power. It was inhabited by the memories of all of the dead of the past and Jung believed that these voices were the source of mental illnesses. This finds echoes in the tendency of different religions to offer prayers for the dead in the hope that they rest in peace.

Roman Catholics, prone to mythology and symbolism, have developed affinities with Jung, although not without controversy. Jung believed that Catholics, in psychoanalysis, needed to be reconciled within their Church before healing could be complete and the transference resolved. Largely, this was because Jung extended the 'desires' of the unconscious (via the transference) towards a Godhead, which transcended the therapist. Jung surmised that this happened in confession, the priest becoming a vessel into which people poured their fears and misgivings. King (1999) connects this process of (transferential) healing to a phrase of St Augustine's: 'You have made us for yourself, O God, and our hearts are restless until they find their rest in you.' It was Jung's view that people become neurotic not because of the irritant of sexual repression but because of the inexpressibility of their religious instinct. His view was that enlightenment came through discovering the meaning of symbols derived from the collective unconscious: his inquiries extended beyond Christianity and he took the notion of the 'numinous' from Eastern religion. This is an intuitive sense of a power that is present but intangible and it is central to religious experience: it *is* religious experience. Ironically, it sits awkwardly with much of post-Enlightenment analytic theology while forming the basis for what passes as person-centred or humanistic therapies. These therapies derive their power from assumptions about the inherent goodness (of man) and the creation of a therapeutic arena composed of acceptance, non-judgementalism and empathy: a kind of playground of the emotions wherein an attempt is made to create a sense of what may or may not be true. The question now becomes: how does this approach bear down on the processes and structures of confession? For example, should penitents derive psychological sustenance from confessing in addition to acquiring discipline and forbearance?

> We must begin with a truism: if deviants are to be corrected they must not be indefinably isolated or alienated. They must obviously be reformed, reconciled, and integrated. To have a method of condemnation without a way to forgive and restore would be self-defeating.
>
> Tentler (1977: 347–348)

In effect, a tension arises between confession as either adjudication or psychological comfort. If confession instils awe and spiritual deference in its supplicants, so too does this reassure them that its sacramental structure is appropriate to the saving power it represents. The accusation is that confessors have strayed too far from this spiritual camp in their eagerness to assume a counselling/caring function. Professor Michael Garanzini (1998: i) says:

> There can be no more challenging situation for the Christian Churches, especially for the Roman Catholic Church, than bringing our theology of healing and reconciliation up to par with contemporary thought on how relationships develop, grow, fail, and sometimes repair themselves.

By contemporary thought he means social and cultural analysis, what he sees as the importance of 'healing and reparation in human relationships, especially as described by humanists and relational psychologists' (p. ii). The implication is clear: relationships point to a renewal of confession as reconciliation not just between the individual and God, but also as part of a social project aimed at ecumenical renewal and making the church once again coterminous with the children of God. For Perrin (1998), this represents a 'new beginning', where sacramental confession rests not only on 'theological, juridical or historical grounds, but on anthropological and existential grounds as well'. By existentialist is meant that we account for the creation of the universe but find meaning within creation as individuals in partnership with humanity. As such, confession should not:

> have as its focus the discernment of guilt and the *mere* (my italics) telling of 'sin'. In the Sacrament of Reconciliation the human person, ultimately, confronts the limits of his or her own life in a humanising way that ought to enhance human freedom for action at both the personal and communal levels.
>
> Perrin (1998: 7)

Here, he distinguishes between ecclesiastically contrived lists of sins to which penitents match their behaviour, and the evolution of personal norms and values 'nurtured through one's faith journey'. In the latter, rules are internalized by individuals and their violation induces existential loss or abandonment. In the older sense of sins – as categories enunciated by traditional churches – one confessed to things external to the self and, in this case, true reconciliation supposedly becomes difficult because the penitent is cast in the role of passive recipient. Perrin (1998: 115) refers to Eliade (1969), who says that 'we are always in the process of appropriating who we are', and at that point the overlap with Rogerian ideas (Rogers, 1951) is blatant. Rogers talked of people stuck, unable to achieve 'organismic whole', and his response to this is based pointedly on empathy. Whatever the transgressions of the client, these must be viewed holistically, and judgement must not cloud his natural progression towards growth and self-actualization. The following (Perrin, 1998: 116) illustrates the point of comparison:

> The ambiguity and fragility of the human condition must first be recognised. This ambiguity and fragility shows itself in *what we refer to as sin* (my italics), but sin is not the mere transgression of pre-determined laws as has already been stated. If this were the case it would be relatively simple to overcome sin by righting the wrong act in as much as this was possible in any particular circumstances. However, it is only through a natural and gradual process of maturation that sin is healed and we are inclined not to sin again. It is this healing which actually thrusts the individual into a greater fullness and appreciation of life. Human fragility can thus become our greatest strength.

Later, Perrin (1998: 133) talks of the priest as 'companion and not judge, helping the penitent discover his or her freedom to choose'.

Problems

There are problems with this at both practical and theological levels. Writers like Perrin concede that their form of reconciliation takes time, and so one wonders how, with fewer and fewer priests, one could engage with penitents in such a protracted way. Further, what evidence is there that people *want* forms of reconciliation which are indistinguishable from counselling? Perhaps what is intended, particularly in the desire to reinvent communal absolution, is a means of obtaining fulfilment by externalizing 'conflicts' and generally 'sharing' in the style of group therapy?

Also, how can human fragility (identified as 'what we refer to as sin') be our greatest strength? In what way is sin strength? I was brought up to avoid sinning at all costs; one even had to shun 'occasions of sin' situations or circumstances where sin would be more rather than less likely to occur.

> For a man is for the moost parte condicioned euen lyke unto them that he kepeth company wythe ...
>
> Bullinger (1541)

Of course, these were the typical sins of the sort listed in the Catechism, what Perrin calls 'the mere transgression of pre-determined laws', and, true, these sins could be said to originate outside the person. Yet such sins bear a remarkable resemblance to the kinds of sins one *liked* to commit, and this, I think, is a problem for 'new (existentialist) theology', which misses the point that ecclesiastical lists of sins are not formulated in a vacuum, but tap into collective agreements of what constitutes sin and, especially, the benefits that sinning brings. Always aware that he continues to enjoy that which sin has gained him, Shakespeare's Claudius cries out:

> May one be pardon'd and retain the offence?
>
> From *Hamlet* (Shakespeare, 1994: III, iii, l.56)

It would appear not. In addition to penance, reparation must be made wherever possible and Claudius (ll.61–66) knows that, in heaven:

> There is no shuffling, there the action lies
> In his true nature; and we ourselves compell'd,

Even to the teeth and forehead of our faults,
To give in evidence. What then? What rests?
Try what repentance can: what can it not?
Yet what can it when one can not repent?

Try as we might, pangs of conscience thwart rationalizing or imagining sins away. Yet in a post-Freudian world, confessors need to know what may lie behind a sinner's narrative; whether, for instance, excessive scrupulousness is a product of depression. Suspecting this, a confessor should heed the Pope's advice and refer the penitent elsewhere. However, typically the issue is not mental illness but more a question of whether confessed sins are violations of God's laws, or if instead, or in addition to, they stem from psychological doubt, misgivings or diminished self-esteem. It seems hard to see – given what Ramon (1985) calls 'the psychologisation of everyday life' – how religion can resist counselling or interpersonal approaches to pastoral care. Indeed, psychological techniques have now transformed our lives so that even those who are not psychologists find that their professional relationships with others are governed by psychological thinking and its correlates.

So does this mean that confession is a psychological technique to restore unhappy people to happiness? Sixty years ago, Hocking noticed psychologists' attempts to set up a subjective equivalent for religion:

> Thus, the cure of souls proceeds on findings of psychiatry ... in lofty disregard of the supernaturalism of traditional religion: psychology will thus put religion on a scientific basis. The proffered help of the Buddha or of the Christ may be graciously declined, for 'salvation' now means 'integration' or 'release' or 'sublimation' and the confessional is simplified into a technical self-disgorgery.
>
> Hocking (1976: 34)

Hocking's doubts are still relevant: contemporary psychotherapies and/or psychologies of the self seem little different from older preoccupations with the soul – as Jung pointed out. If one takes a concept from Rogerian theory such as 'organismic' – the quality of individuals organizing themselves towards wholeness and ultimate goodness – nowhere is the concept defined with any greater scientific specificity than that. Thinly disguised as some kind of scientific description, it amounts to little more than an article of faith. For Hocking:

> The omission of the religious object does not do. Modern man ... must resume connection with his soul, and what, pray, is that? It is simply the self, concerned with its realities, its objects of widest scope, its absolutes. The self cannot be cut off from its object, as a state of mind, and remain anything at all.
>
> Hocking (1976: 34)

This, of course, is an affirmation of faith: outside of faith it is merely the substitution of one word, 'soul', for another, 'self'. In fact, as psychological concepts go, the 'self' is problematic: from Ryle's (1963) *The Concept of Mind* to more contemporary accounts (see Howard, 2001), the self, from the point of view of empirical or analytic inquiry, is not an invincible idea. And yet we'd be lost without it. It bears down on the question of free will, which we must have if we are to commit sins. Because if 'merely' at the mercy of a Freudian unconscious, if merely the product of day-to-day behavioural stimuli, or if merely an epiphenomenon of our neurobiology, we are hardly accountable for or to anything. For accountability to occur there must be an 'us', which directs what we do, and this has to be an immaterial force of some kind (see Magee, 2000: 569–573). Such a force is not synonymous with religious belief but it is central to religion and it makes sense of faith, of the hope of salvation. Many philosophers, of course, would see assertions about an immaterial force as discarding reason, as a flight into fable and allegory, useful as instruments of argumentation but not much more. But, for many, cowardice and conscience go hand in hand and religion becomes the milieu where this is made sense of and articulated through faith and confessing one's sins *as sins*. Undeniably, psychological comfort will come from this. However, a profounder consolation may flow from the (difficult) belief that sacred forgiveness for wrongs actually committed is possible. Transforming sins into frailty deprives us of our autonomy: it implies that we cannot (always) assume responsibility for our actions. Alternatively, sacramental confession challenges us to accept responsibility, to look at how our actions bring about gratification and aggrandisement, and accept penance and retribution both as punishment and verification of sovereign agency.

References

Bullinger H (1541) The Christian State of Matrimonye (translated by M Coverdale). Antwerp: J Hoochstraten (reprinted 1974).

Dostoyevsky F (1951) Crime and Punishment. Harmondsworth: Penguin.

Eliade M (1969) The Quest: history and meaning in religion. Chicago: University of Chicago Press.

Fordham F (1953) An Introduction to Jung's Psychology. London: Penguin.

Foucault M (1999) Religion and Culture. Manchester: Manchester University Press.

Garanzini MJ (1998) Foreword. In: Perrin DB (ed.) The Sacrament of Reconciliation: an existentialist approach. New York: The Edwin Mellen Press.

Graham AC (1971) Confucianism. In: Zaehner RC (ed.) The Concise Encyclopaedia of Living Faiths, 2nd edn, pp. 357–373. London: Hutchinson.

Hobbes T (1909) Leviatian. Oxford: Clarendon Press (reprinted from 1651 edn).

Hocking WE (1976) Living Religions and a World Faith. New York: Macmillan.

Howard A (2001) Fallacies and realities of self. Community Psychiatry Journal May: 19–23.

John Paul II (1994) Crossing the Bridges of Hope. London: Jonathan Cape.

King TM (1999) Jung's Four and Some Philosophers: a paradigm for philosophy. Indiana: Notre Dame Press.

Magarshack D (1951) Introduction. In: Crime and Punishment (Dostoyevsky F). Harmondsworth: Penguin.

Magee B (2000) Confessions of a Philosopher: a journey through Western philosophy. London: Phoenix Books.

Nelson B (1965) Self images and systems of spiritual direction in the history of European civilisation. In: Klausner S (ed.) The Quest for Self Control. New York: Free Press.

Noss JB (1974) Man's Religions, 5th edn. London: Collier Macmillan.

O'Dea JK, O'Dea TF, Adams CT (1972) Judaism, Christianity and Islam. London: Harper & Row.

O'Grady P (2002) Relativism. Chesham, Bucks: Acumen Publishing.

O'Loughlin T (2000) Celtic Theology. London: Continuum.

Perrin DB (1998) The Sacrament of Reconciliation: an existential approach. Lewiston, New York: The Edwin Mellen Press.

Peters M http://faculty.ed.uiuc.edu/burbules/ncb/syllabi/Materials/Confession.html

Pless JT (2001) Your pastor is not your therapist: private confession – the ministry of repentance and faith. In: A Reader in Pastoral Theology, pp. 92–102. Fort Wayne, IN: Concordia Theological Seminary Press.

Ramon S (1985) Psychiatry in Britain. Beckenham: Croom Helm.

Rausch T (1998) Sexual morality and social justice. In: Heyes MA and Gearon L (eds) Contemporary Catholic Theology: a reader, pp. 403–433. Leominster, Herts: Gracewing.

Rogers C (1951) Client-centred Therapy: its current practice, implications and theory. London: Constable.

Rose N (1989) Governing the Soul: the shaping of the private self. London: Routledge.

Ryle G (1963) The Concept of Mind. Harmondsworth: Penguin.

Shakespeare W (1994) The Complete Works of William Shakespeare. London: HarperCollins.

Tambling J (1990) Confession: sexuality, sin, the subject. Manchester: Manchester University Press.

Tentler TN (1977) Sin and Confession on the Eve of the Reformation. Princeton, NJ: Princeton University Press.

Wittgenstein L (1953) Philosophical Investigations. Oxford: Blackwell.

Zernov N (1971) Christianity: the Eastern Schism and the Eastern Orthodox Church. In: Zaehner RC (ed.) The Concise Encyclopaedia of Living Faiths, 2nd edn, pp. 77–93. London: Hutchinson.

CHAPTER 8
Pilgrimage

EIBHLIN INGLESBY

Eibhlin Inglesby has been a nurse and has taught nursing and theology. She is now primarily a carer of various generations of family members and tries to make sense of life while doing so.

The journey

In some respects, the notion of pilgrimage as a metaphor for life's exterior and interior journeying is an obvious one, trite almost. A pilgrimage is usually conceived of as a journey to a sacred or very special place. It is a well-known phenomenon within all the major world religions and indeed appears to have been a fundamental activity from the earliest times. Even in a secular age, people freely use the term pilgrimage to describe a journey of significance, whether it be to Diana's funeral, in support of football heroes or the search for one's biological or national roots. Pilgrimage is a journey with a goal in mind, a purposeful activity.

It seems to me that this is the point where the analogy with life begins to fall away. One can, of course, see the concept of time going by as the steps of a journey. But what do we mean when we talk of purpose or (sacred) goals in life? There are other discrepancies: classical pilgrimage also involves a return journey back from the 'sacred' to the 'mundane' world. The pilgrim must be penitent and prepared to endure (if not seek out) hardship. Medieval Christian pilgrims often sold or gave up all they owned prior to embarking on the journey and made wills and provisions for their families, because it was quite likely that they would not return, so great were the dangers of travel. The more one investigates its intricacies, the less pilgrimage may appear to be a meaningful metaphor; one that should perhaps only be used superficially. I would like to suggest, however, that it is

such intricacies (and many more) that make pilgrimage a rich and therapeutic symbol, one worthy of investigation and contemplation. I will
therefore try to describe more fully these intricacies in order to discuss their
relationship to our spiritual, mental and physical wellbeing.

The anthropologist Victor Turner described pilgrimage as extroverted
mysticism and mysticism as introverted pilgrimage (Turner and Turner,
1975: 33). This is neat and in some ways helpful, but fails to grasp the
key element that a journey becomes a pilgrimage precisely because of
both interior *and* exterior movement. One may physically travel for many
obvious reasons. Interior travel appears more complex but need not be;
academic inquiry, meditation, fantasy, distress, poetry, psychosis – all
involve interior journeying, sometimes helpful, sometimes not. The
point of pilgrimage is, however, that it does not merely combine the two
journeys but rather synthesizes them so that thoughts and steps necessi-
tate each other. It involves mental, physical and spiritual integrity. In
other words, it is like life. But to be too enigmatic is not necessarily to be
helpful and to give illustrations of pilgrims and their journeys might be
more so.

Practice

Historically, pilgrimage[1] has been practised in what seems to be different
ways. There has been the 'popular' journeying to a holy place for a special purpose, often a journey of intercession for an important request, or
as a penance (a way of showing and not just saying that one is sorry) for
an act regretted – a way of trying to access that which is greater than ourselves in times of crisis. What is interesting is the universal notion that this
access will come by leaving (physically) one's normal environment in
order to journey to another 'realm'. Anthropologists (and some religious
commentators) are inclined to describe this as a move from the 'mundane' to the 'sacred', as if there were some borderline or frontier which
led from one to the other. Indeed, the notion of a veil between the mundane and the sacred is a universally recognized religious symbol. Celtic
Christianity described a holy place as one where the veil is more transparent and thus reveals the sacred more clearly. This veil is not just a
visual phenomenon but one which mediates or blocks total experience,
so at a holy place one not only 'sees' more clearly but also 'feels' more
accurately the whole of existence.

However one might interpret the world and our place in it, most people appear to recognize that some places just do feel different and that

---

[1]   My descriptions will be of Christian pilgrimage, because it is the area that I know best.
    I suspect that much of what is said would apply throughout the major religions.

some places make *us* feel different about ourselves and life around us. It is also a general wisdom that sometimes one has to leave normal everyday life in order to experience life itself more fully – get out of a rut, a change is as good as a rest. There may be many explanations for this phenomenon but few of us will not recognize it.

There are also problems with this view of reality. Why, we may ask, if we have physical, mental and spiritual integrity, should existence be divided into the mundane (or secular) and the sacred? Why is our experience of life so apparently fragmented? Theologians and psychologists have abundant answers to this dilemma, some more satisfactory than others. It was also a problem that made a difference to the way some pilgrims thought of themselves. In the early centuries of the Christian religion, some believers decided that the only way to find the truth of themselves and their God was to isolate themselves, in every sense from the world as they knew it, by going into exile in the desert, to literally live in a wilderness landscape in the hope that 'being nowhere' and 'being no one' would give them a clue to their real identity. These people are generally referred to as the Desert Fathers, but there were women too. The reasoning, thoughts and practices which informed their lives are not always comfortable reading, for there was a sense in which the world and life was seen as evil and a distraction to the true path.[2] However, what must be noted is that these believers considered themselves to be pilgrims not merely because they had travelled from the city to the desert, but because they had renounced the identity with which they had been endowed by the world. They preferred to live with the uncertainty of no identity until they understood who they really were. That was the essence of being a pilgrim.

Seeking spiritual insight

J'aurais voulu Marie des Routes
Emprunter l'un de tes chemins,
Et croiser, au cours de mes doutes,
Le regard de ces pélerins.
Qui dans la nuit et la lumière,
Marchent vers tes sanctuaires

Les circonstances de ma vie
Ne m'appellent pas aux voyages.
Et je peux te trouver aussi
Sur les chemins de mon village,
Au hazard des rencontres de l'été,
Dans quelques paroles échangées.

---

[2] This view has persisted in some understandings of Christianity and was much later adopted in a more moderate fashion by Bunyan in the *Pilgrim's Progress.*

Marie des ruisseaux et terrents,
Marie des cascades puissantes,
Marie du soleil levant,
Derrière les cimes imposantes,
Marie des luminuex matins,
Marie des menaçants orages,
Marie du vent dans sapins,
Marie du parfum des alpages,
Marie du vol majesteux,
Fais-nous connaître la trace
Des chemins qui mènent à Dieu.

À travers tous les paysages,
Je ferai mon pélerinage.

(See chapter appendix for translation)

I saw this poem/prayer in the church of Marie de Santé in Carcassonne in southwest France, which had been and still is a stopping-off point along the Camino or Route St Jacques. The Camino leads to Santiago de Compostela, a town in northwest Spain that has been the object of pilgrimage for a thousand years. The poem is perhaps slightly anarchistic because, while honouring those who travel traditional pilgrim routes, it suggests that they are only one means to spiritual insight. The writer says most beautifully and vividly that the sacred may be beheld in the extraordinary nature of creation and indeed of everyday life. Pilgrimage has become something different again. It is a way of encountering what may be thought of as the mundane, and seeing it as a reflection of the holy.

Moreover, one feels that the writer is not only expressing an objective sense of wonder but also confirming her identity as part of that wonder. We seem to have moved from a temporary physical journey to the sacred; to removing oneself totally to a place where the sacred may be sought; to being able to view the sacred in one's everyday world. The Christian Celts had moved in this latter direction, having been inspired by the Desert Fathers. They believed that God was revealed in creation and thus accessible anywhere, but the trap lay in becoming tied to human structures of power. Many Celtic saints thus saw their vocation as pilgrims as one of perpetual wandering. If one place is potentially as holy as another, there can be no destination of significance. The understanding of one's identity comes not with the question 'Who am I?', but with the question 'Where am I?'. One's relationship with the journey somehow forms and reveals the truth.

Paths to salvation

It is not easy to tie all these threads together. What can be distilled from these varying interpretations of pilgrimage that will make a coherent theme? In whichever way it has been interpreted, movement appears to be essential: whether it be a series of sporadic journeys, a total exiling, a constant movement of interpretation within a fixed landscape, or wandering in ever new landscapes. Pilgrimage seems to tell us that to be 'fixed' is a form of spiritual death.

Even if the movement has no apparent physical goal it is not aimless. It advocates a form of homelessness in order to find one's real home. St Jerome was scathing of those who undertook long pilgrimages to Jerusalem believing that the physical action alone would help them: 'It will not benefit you to journey to Jerusalem if you do not have Jerusalem in your heart' (Sumption, 1975: 101). The Celtic saints believed that they carried the heavenly Jerusalem within them. These people lived with metaphors that may be totally meaningless to us, but what they were really discussing was the search for meaning and identity in their lives. For them it lay in relationship to the God that they perceived. The symbols and metaphors may need changing, but the wisdom remains the same: in order to find out who you really are you need to leave everything behind and, in losing yourself, you will find the answer to that paradoxical question of identity. Pilgrimage not only gives a verbal wisdom but also translates it into a way of being – a way of constantly 'being' on the move.

Still, of course, we encounter problems. I have never been able to reconcile myself to Bunyan's hero, Pilgrim, who is prepared to leave his wife and family in order to follow the straight and narrow path to salvation. It seems so fundamentally uncharitable. Bunyan's tale may be better read as a parable than as an allegory, but it still gives the feeling that movement towards personal enlightenment may involve a shunning of one's other responsibilities. Being on the move can sometimes be an awful lot easier than staying put. This is not what pilgrimage is advocating. It was never seen as the easy option. St Colmcille, it is said, exiled himself from his native Donegal as a penance for starting a war. Hundreds of people walk an arduous and dangerous route for hundreds of miles to Santiago de Compostela to prove that they are earnest in their search. Penance and a sense of ascetic hardship are generally alien concepts these days, often associated with an outdated and gratuitously sadistic notion of religious truth. The age of 'supermarket' spirituality, where you can pick and choose what you like and leave behind what you don't, is definitely with us. The point that seems to be missed is that while pointless suffering is undoubtedly wrong, there are some paths in life in which suffering may

be unavoidable, if one is insistent on reaching the other side. All movement carries with it the risk of danger and hardship.

Nor does pilgrimage necessarily suggest that exile alone holds the key.
Jimmy Boyle, who was imprisoned for murder, had spent years in solitary
confinement. He was then moved to a more modern and social prison system where he was made to confront and come to terms with his previous
crimes. The second prison was much more comfortable and humane in
every way, but he relates that initially he would have given anything to be
back in solitary confinement (in a fixed psychological place) rather than
go through the journey to his new sense of identity. He realized on this
journey that he could not be remade unless he was entirely broken first.
He described that process as excruciating, but unavoidable and ultimately life saving.

Thus, by movement, I am suggesting many things: physical, metaphorical, mental and sensory. The Jesuit theologian Michel de Certeau also
suggested its importance as a political phenomenon. He considered it the
duty of the Christian (who is always a pilgrim in a sense) to be constantly on the move, never residing in places of power but always living in the
interstices of society, in the 'spaces' between the places. He advocated a
resistant practice of living that challenged all boundaries. The work of pilgrimage as a symbol of Christian life thus becomes a constant shifting of
the goalposts, a movement from places of power, which we may have
come to call home or nation or self, into the space beyond. This 'space'
might be seen as a kind of no-man's-land or wilderness, a landscape that
allows for constant redefinition of one's being.

Madness as salvation?

I have tried to describe what I see as the complex nature of pilgrimage,
which, although simply summed up as 'a journey to a holy place', is in fact
a rich metaphorical image if one moves creatively within the concepts
involved. The theme of this book is, however, spirituality and mental
health, and I must now endeavour to bridge what may appear to be the
gaps between my understanding of pilgrimage as a spiritual guideline,
and its application to notions of mental wellbeing. I can only really do this
by putting my cards on the table. Like everyone else I speak from a stance
of belief, which informs the way I view human being and identity, as well
as our relationship to the world around us and to its other inhabitants.
Broadly speaking that belief involves the existence of something greater
than ourselves, in which our true identity and purpose lies. But this relationship of meaning is not simply a 'vertical' one between us as
individuals and the Other; it is also a horizontal one between us and other

individuals and creatures and our environment. Our identity can thus be seen as relational, both intrinsically in our existence as biological, psychological, social and spiritual beings, and extrinsically in our relationship to the world around us. Pilgrimage, in its necessary coupling of the physical with the mental, seems entirely apt as a symbol of the integration necessary for us to be mentally well. There is more to it than this, of course. Mental distress so often appears to involve problems of identity, either because we do not know who we really are or because our sense of who we are is not accepted by others as valid. The religious or spiritual quest is often associated with the word salvation, which in turn has popularly been connected to ideas of an afterlife. But salvation may mean many things:

Every old man I see
Reminds me of my father
When he had fallen in love with death
One time when sheaves were gathered.

That man I saw in Gardner St.
Stumble on the kerb was one
He stared at me half-eyed
I might have been his son.

And I remember the musician
Faltering over his fiddle
In Bayswater, London
He too set me the riddle.

Every old man I see
In October-coloured weather
Seems to say to me
'I was once your father.'

                                                                    Patrick Kavanagh

As he wandered through anonymous cities, did the poet search faces on park benches, in doorways, under arches – the homeless homes of those whose identity is lost – in the hope of finding the place where he, himself, might at last come to rest, subsumed in the visage of another? Does he epitomize the wandering pilgrim in all of us? Salvation may be as 'simple' as being 'found', feeling safe, feeling an extraordinary sense of peace. But for many of us that will involve a lot of travelling and a lot of searching and probably no little hardship.

There are records through the ages of a special type of pilgrim who came to be known as 'holy fool'. The tradition is particularly associated with the Near East in the early centuries of Christianity, and with Russia from the Middle Ages to the 19th century. These characters made a life's work of being outrageous. They would wander scantily clothed even in the height of winter, tending the sick, provoking the rich, protesting about state and social injustices, and preaching the gospel. St Simeon Salos (translated as Simon the Crackpot) was famous for being even more outlandish. He entered churches and threw nuts at women present, dressed outrageously, exhibited violent mood swings, publicly ate sausages on Good Friday and on one occasion entered a public bath reserved only for women. At the end of his life, however, he confided that he had done all of these acts as an expression of *apathea* or passionlessness. He had made himself 'mad' in order to be an outcast, for only as such could he live the life of private prayer that he sought as the expression of his true identity (Saward, 1980: 19–20).

In our 'enlightened', 'tolerant', postmodern world, which refuses to privilege one story over another, we have, however, no space, and only one place for the holy fool. Whether his madness was simulated or not, Simeon would probably be diagnosed ('classical' schizophrenic symptoms), incarcerated and 'treated'. However, such incarceration, although putting an end to his physical pilgrim wanderings, would not have thwarted his real aim. For his real aim was the extreme desire of the pilgrim, not only to possess *nothing* and to be *nowhere* but also to be *nobody*.

What, you may quite legitimately ask, can the somewhat dubious antics of a fourth-century dissident have to do with our everyday striving to have a place in the world? I appear to be condemning all who search for the truth either to an exterior wilderness or an interior madness. The journey so far seems to be one of dissemblance, what de Certeau calls the 'broken I'. What pilgrimage tells us, is that it is that very desire for a 'place' to inhabit that may well be the cause of the distress. 'Places' are constructs of human power and control. They do not help us to find reality but separate us from it by enforced conformity to what is, after all, merely a reality constructed by others. To be a pilgrim is to search out the 'spaces', where the veil is most transparent and we have room to be who we are meant to be. For those whose 'confinement' (whether it be physical or metaphorical or both) causes them mental distress, the notion of pilgrimage offers a trajectory of hope. It does not promise an easy ride but it does offer possibility.

To be a pilgrim

At the beginning I mentioned sacred goals and asked how we can find out what these are. The answer that pilgrimage gives to this is rather like a Zen riddle. The 'true' pilgrim (as opposed to the 'spiritual tourist') does not know wherein lies her destination. Even those who journey to specific places have only a mental marker before them. Pilgrims always travel into the unknown. Their true destination is uncertain. Pilgrimage is an act of faith that does not renounce responsibilities to others but which leaves behind harmful and binding structures.

There are no direct corollaries between mental health and pilgrimage. I believe that the very great distress caused by depression is (to use a somewhat medieval phrase) a *great sadness of the soul*. It feels like spiritual death because one feels trapped in a life where movement has become impossible. To leave such a place one has to travel through the darkness into uncertainty. The truth is that not everyone does find light at the end of that darkness, but that is not because the light is not there. It may be because there have been no friendly hands or resting posts along the way. Nonetheless, I am convinced that depression can be a pilgrimage; an arduous journey in which one must be prepared to be broken in order to live again (or indeed in some cases to live for the first time).

Most people can understand depression or anxiety and many of the other myriad so-called neurotic disorders. Madness (or psychosis, its sanitized label) is a much more perplexing phenomenon. Madness has always had a bad press, although 'Christ's Madmen' (the holy fools) were probably tolerated better than most. People fear madness for many reasons. Sometimes this is because mad people behave in threatening or aggressive ways. Most people whose behaviour is hostile to others are not mad, however. They are considered sane, culpable and probably 'bad'. Yet all manifestations of madness are likely to be vilified and feared because it leaves the boundaries of 'safety' and sets out on an unknown journey of exploration. It would be foolishly romantic to suggest that all journeys of madness are pilgrimages. One imagines that some are experiences of hell. But the sane can experience hell too. There are good and bad journeys for all. What we should not negate, however, is the potential of a journey in madness to be a holy one, for after all it does have the classic characteristics of true pilgrimage.

No single metaphor can explain to us the meaning of our lives. To think of ourselves as pilgrims in many ways provides no answer, but it might point us in the right direction on a road to discovery. Classical literature usually speaks of that road as a 'straight and narrow' one, and I have emphasized that one must expect difficulties to arise, but the straight and narrow always seems a shade unimaginative as a pathway in such a gloriously diverse world. Personally, like Robert Frost, I would prefer to 'take the road less travelled' or meander like my Celtic ancestors. Although there is bound to be hardship there is no prohibition on enjoyment, particularly if one allows the road itself to inform the journey. In Herman Hesse's (1982) masterpiece, Siddhartha the ferryman and the river become one, so harmonious has their journey become.

I have used the word 'place' in a negative sense as a position of con-
striction. That is not to confuse it with the idea of a landscape, physical or
metaphorical. It is our interaction with these landscapes that allows us to
be pilgrims. In talking of the physical world Simon Schama writes, 'Before
it can ever be a repose for the senses, landscape is the work of the mind.
Its scenery is built up as much from strata of memory as from layers of
rock' (Schama, 1995: 6). Morley and Robins in turn make a similar link,
suggesting that identity is 'a question of memory and memories of home
in particular' (Morley and Robins, 1995: 10). I feel that both of these state-
ments are true and that it is the memory of where we have been that tells
us not only who we are, but where we are. Pilgrimage takes us further
along the road by giving us memories of the future, of a future home; and
when we begin to live those memories it may be that the questions 'Who
am I?' or even 'Where am I?' will no longer need an answer:

> Until one is committed, there is hesitancy, the chance to draw back, always
> ineffectiveness ... that moment one commits oneself, then providence
> moves all. All sorts of things occur to help one that would never have
> otherwise occurred. A whole stream of events issues from the decision,
> raising in one's favour all manner of unseen incidents and meetings and
> material assistance which no man would have dreamed could have come his
> way. Whatever you can do or dream you can, begin it. Boldness has genius,
> power and magic in it. Begin it now.
>
> Goethe (quoted in Goss, 1999)

Begin the journey now.

References

Goss P (1999) Close to the Wind. London: Headline Press, p. 114.
Hesse H (1982) Siddhartha. NY: Bantam Books.
Morley D and Robins K (1995) Spaces of Identity. London: Routledge.
Saward J (1980) Perfect Fools. Oxford: Oxford University Press.
Schama S (1995) Landscape and Memory. London: Fontana Press.
Sumption J (1975) Pilgrimage: an image of medieval religion. London: Faber and
    Faber.
Turner V and Turner E (1975) Image and Pilgrimage in Christian Culture. New
    York: Columbia University Press.

Recommended reading

Carter E, Donald J and Squires J (1993) Space and Place Theories of Identity and
    Location. London: Lawrence and Wishart.

Coleman S and Elsner J (1995) Pilgrimage: past and present in world religions. London: British Museum Press.

de Certeau M (1988) The Practice of Everyday Life. London: University of California Press.

de Certeau M (1995) The Mystic Fable. Chicago: University of Chicago Press.

Eade J and Salnow M (1991) Contesting the Sacred. London: Routledge.

Appendix

Seeking spiritual insight (translation)

I would have liked, Mary of the pathways
To follow one of your roads
And in the midst of my doubts
To meet your pilgrims
Who travel night and day to your sanctuaries.

The circumstances of life
Have not called upon me to journey
But I can find you
In the roads of my own village
In the chance meetings of summertime
In conversations exchanged

Mary of the streams and torrents
Mary of the cascading waterfalls
Mary of the sun that rises behind the resplendent peaks
Mary of glittering mornings
Mary of menacing storms
Mary of the wind in the trees
Mary of the sweet smelling pastures
Mary of majestic birds in flight
Make known to us the outlines of roads that lead to God

My journey through every landscape will be my pilgrimage.

CHAPTER 9
Discipline

SALLY CLAY

Sally Clay recovered from severe mental illness through the practice of Tibetan Buddhism. She has been a leader in the mental health consumer/survivor movement in the USA for over 20 years, and is Executive Editor of a book in progress called *Doing It Our Way: peer programs that work for people with mental illness*. She works as consultant to the Triad Women and Violence Project in Florida. She previously worked for Windhorse Associates, an alternative treatment programme, and helped to found four consumer-run services: the Portland Coalition in Maine, PEOPLe in upstate New York, the PEER Center in Florida and Altered States of the Arts. Her writings are posted on ZANGMO BLUE THUNDER-CLOUD (http://home.earthlink.net/~sallyclay).

Beginnings

Spirituality was both the cause of my madness and its cure. From an early age I sought out spiritual experiences, sometimes known as altered states. These became both the basis of my faith and the trigger of mental illness.

Years before my first mental breakdown I defined my life and beliefs by a night in Colorado during the summer of my sixteenth year. I was on an overnight trip with girls from my summer camp, and we spent the night beside a high mountain lake called Loch Vale. Unable to sleep, I dragged my sleeping bag onto a big rock at the side of the lake, where I sat alone and instinctively adopted a meditative position with crossed legs and erect posture. I sat all night in the silence of wilderness with only the light of the stars reflecting in the lake and silhouetting the three black mountains on the other side. At first my thoughts jumped about, with worries about problems at home. Then, becoming more aware of the landscape

122

around me, I thought self-consciously about what I labelled the 'beauty of nature' and the 'glory of God'. At some point in the middle of the night my thoughts stopped altogether, and my mind filled with a refreshing emptiness. This altered state was not a dramatic realization but a matter-of-fact clarity and peace. I was still aware of my surroundings, but the lake, the mountains, the air were no longer separate from me. I felt transparent. Eventually the black clarity gave way to a grey light creeping over the mountains, and conventional reality returned with the dawn.

At the time, I did not consider my experience to be a big deal. I had always enjoyed what I called 'communing with nature' – spending time sitting outdoors by streams or lakes. The experience at Loch Vale seemed nothing unusual. I did, however, puzzle that I had sat for so long with no thoughts at all, and I even wondered if there was, perhaps, something wrong with me! It had never occurred to me that consciousness without thoughts was possible, much less desirable. Gradually, as I returned to everyday life and high school, I began to appreciate the significance of my experience, and even wrote about it, because it seemed to mark a turning point in my life – from child to adult, from doubter to believer. On Sundays I began arriving early at church so that I could stay a long time on my knees, not mouthing prayers but evoking the inner silence that I had found in the mountains. What I had discovered, I later learned, was what Buddhists call 'emptiness', the foundation of spiritual realization.

Spiritual breakthrough

College was stressful. Since the age of seven I had called myself a writer, but now I was faced with the prospect of having to earn a living. I felt alienated from society and even from friends and family, and any writing I attempted seemed self-conscious rather than creative. I felt somehow different from everybody else, and inadequate. Nevertheless, I plodded along conscientiously until the middle of my junior year, when life blew up on me.

It started with another spiritual experience, this one dramatic and overwhelming. I sat in my dorm room listening to a recording of TS Eliot reading his own *Four Quartets*. His funereal words, 'Time present and time past, are both perhaps present in time future', took on meanings beyond poetry and became to me instructions in Universal Truth. I felt the boundaries of time dissolve, leaving me at the still point that was the convergence of the ultimate and the particular.

My altered state three years before in Colorado had been clear and quiet. This one was filled with colour and energy. Thoughts, associations and every visual object leapt and danced together, all leading to luminosity and joy, and an exquisite appreciation of all things. Now, 40 years later, it is still impossible to describe this state adequately. I believed then, and still do believe, that I had encountered true reality, the solution to a great secret which, in essence, was that all things are interconnected and all things are beautiful. In this condition, my body was not transparent, as it had been by the lake, but transformed. I found that I could lift heavy objects with no strain, and my senses were sharpened – for example, I could see clearly without the use of my glasses. This was the beginning of my first manic episode, an experience, I suppose, of what the doctors call 'elation'. But this state should not be pathologized. I was to spend the next three decades trying to recapture that luminosity. It was only when I finally encountered Buddhism that I learned to understand what it all meant and what to do about it.

The brilliance of the luminous state lasted only a day or two. Then, like someone who had overindulged in wine or drugs, I fell into a nightmare of delusion and anguish, and the luminosity disintegrated. I went for days without eating or sleeping, and my mind careened out of control. I drove my friends wild with worry, and when one of them tried to talk me sensibly, I struck her. Finally I was carried off to a mental hospital in an ambulance. Once incarcerated, I was heavily drugged and not once asked to describe the experience that got me there.

Mental and spiritual illness

This was my introduction to a mental health system that enforces its norms with an iron fist, chooses which outcomes to call 'recovery', and conveniently overlooks the mind itself, with all of its spiritual qualities. I stumbled through the next 16 years trying to reach the 'normality' that was required of me, all the while wondering what had really happened in my mind, and secretly yearning to re-experience the joy and colour of that state. Without understanding and incorporating my spiritual experience, my life was unfinished, like the stories I tried to write and could not. Everything I did was doomed to failure.

I married and started to raise two children. But it was not long before I lapsed into one manic episode after another. Although I tried to ride through these episodes with the pleasures and insights of the first one, I was constantly aware that, sooner or later, I would be carried off to the hospital and locked up and drugged. The episodes became recurring nightmares that finally led to admission to a long-term hospital in another state. There I suffered through nearly two years of depression and despair until my husband sued me for divorce, and the hospital released me to live alone, without a home and without my children.

Although I lost custody of my children, I did manage to find satisfying work, first at a printing company, then as a freelance proofreader. I also wrote for the local National Organization of Women newsletter. It was a whole new life for me, and although I experienced more manic episodes, I was able to get through a couple of them alone, with others resulting in hospitalizations of only a few days. Through my feminist activities I met a woman who later became my lover. We bought a house in western Maine, and I took a job as editor and writer for a local newspaper. The mania returned with a vengeance, however, and I lost my job and freaked out my partner with my wild behaviour. She left me alone in the house, and never returned.

Dharma discovered

I had grown up a regular churchgoer, first in the Disciples of Christ church and then as an Episcopalian. I sang in the choirs from an early age and was generally serious and faithful in my Christian beliefs. But after the bouts with madness, I could no longer reconcile my knowledge of luminosity with the Church's teachings. I had long talks with my Episcopal priest, but still could not resolve the issues, or even adequately explain to him what had happened to me. While in Maine, I received instructions from a Christian Science practitioner. I liked a lot of the teachings, although was not persuaded to become a practitioner myself.

But while I worked at the newspaper, I learned that there was a Buddhist meditation centre in Vermont, not too far from us, where a Tibetan lama who had studied at Oxford in England was teaching to American students. One weekend I drove to Karme Chöling, and encountered Chögyam Trungpa, the lama himself, who was just returning from a year-long retreat. Although I did not talk with him personally, I was stunned at the instantaneous connection that I felt. I bought every book that he had written, and was amazed to find that the Buddhist teachings immediately 'fit' with my own beliefs and experiences. Although the Christian teachers that I had consulted about my madness never seemed to understand what I was talking about, the Buddhist writers described in detail mental states very much like the ones I knew, and even gave a name to my experience of luminosity. They called it *mahamudra*, or 'great symbol'.

At Karme Chöling, the principal activity was what was called, simply, 'sitting'. One end of the building was devoted to an enormous shrine room with a polished hardwood floor and decorations in red and gold. Even the meditation cushions were red and gold. I was assigned a meditation instructor, who tried to convince me that the meditation was just 'sitting', and nothing to get excited about. I did not believe her. I already knew what meditation was all about – it was what I had done beside the lake and on the prayer bench in church. I was delighted to find that all of the pieces of my spiritual experience were at last falling into place.

It became frustrating, however, to try to explain myself to the young teachers at Karme Chöling. They were only students themselves, and when I tried to ask about my mental states, they did not seem to know what I was talking about. They seemed to answer by rote, with answers that were 'spiritually correct'. When describing meditation, the students went out of their way to say that it was 'no big deal'. Of course, that was the way that I myself had experienced it. But when the young students described it, they were smug and even flippant, and I felt that they were only mouthing words that they were taught.

Although meditation was 'no big deal', it was practised three times a day, and more often than that during intensive practice sessions. Most of the practitioners seemed to become 'zonked' out after an hour-long session of sitting, but I found it energizing. I had to restrain myself from enthusiastically chatting with others at dinnertime, as the accepted decorum was to maintain a zombie-like mask. It was excruciating to finally encounter the 'truth' but have no one to discuss it with. I did not realize that the more hours I spent in silent meditation, the more my emotions were commandeered by an energy that was not just clarity, but was also the kind of elation that had gotten me in trouble in college. This led to disaster.

I began writing long, intense letters to Rinpoche [Chögyam Trungpa Rinpoche, Sally's first Tibetan teacher], and tried to appear wherever he went, in the hope of obtaining an interview. At one point, in a frenzy of spiritual excitement (and mania), I decided to 'crash' his annual seminary in New Hampshire. I lay in wait for him in the lobby of the hotel, and slipped past his guards to present him with a gift. He had the grace to thank me for it and to ask one of his assistants to give me a room for the night, as it was beginning to snow heavily. I spent the night in a small bedroom on the third floor, looking out at the falling snow that covered the hotel and its environs in deep, white silence. It was almost like a meditation.

I decided that I needed authentic instruction from Tibetan lamas, not from yuppie-like students. Trungpa Rinpoche had spoken of Karma Triyana Dharmachakra (KTD), a new monastery that would become the spiritual home of the Kagyu lineage in America. KTD was located on a mountain road in Woodstock, New York, and after my adventure at the seminary, I drove there. I met three authentic lamas, one of whom was Khenpo Karthar Rinpoche, the abbot. Because the lamas had only recently moved to KTD themselves, there was only a handful of other students.

I was one of only three or four people who took refuge with Khenpo Rinpoche one Sunday afternoon. This ceremony was like a combination of baptism and confirmation. I promised to adhere to and take refuge in 'the Buddha, the Dharma, and the Sangha (community)', without at the same time having to renounce any other religion. Rinpoche gave each of us a Dharma name and a small gift. My name was Karma Tsultrim Zangmo, which I later learned meant 'Member of the Kagyu lineage/Discipline/Good Woman'. I was told that the middle name represented the area in which I had to apply the most effort. I guess I needed discipline!

I was able to arrange for several face-to-face interviews with Khenpo Rinpoche. I spoke to him openly about my mental illness, and my belief that the luminosity I experienced was genuine and meaningful. He accepted this belief of mine (to my astonishment!), but declined to assign a spiritual practice for me, as he did for most of the other students. Instead, he told me that I should take what I had learned from my experience and share it with others in my community. I confess that this disappointed me somewhat, as I had fantasies of diligently praying for several years at the monastery, after which I would reach full enlightenment and become ordained as a nun.

I was still intoxicated with mystical thoughts, and again my energies got the better of me. One night, when all of the lamas were invited to dinner with a Woodstock resident, I became frustrated with the attitude of the other students, who used the lamas' absence to lounge around the living room and speak crudely. On a manic impulse I found the fire alarm in the dining room and broke the glass. The result was awesome. Bells and sirens went off, and a white chemical spilled from the kitchen ceiling and covered everything with a thick white powder. The end result was that the lamas personally escorted me to the sheriff's office, where I was arrested for criminal trespass and sent to jail for a week. Following that I was committed to the state psychiatric hospital in Poughkeepsie, where I spent a miserable, lonely Christmas.

When I returned home to Portland, Maine, I had no clue how to implement Rinpoche's advice to work with other people. My faith in the Dharma remained unshaken, but there was no way to put it into practice. I continued attending the Episcopal Church. I took a job at a radio station and began to attend Alcoholics Anonymous. Reasoning that I drank whenever I got manic, I called myself an alcoholic for two years and enjoyed the system of peer support created by AA. The Twelve Step and Big Book meetings that I attended were helpful, even though I always knew that my problem was not so much that I was powerless over alcohol as it was that I was a prisoner of my mind. As a Buddhist, I never could accept the concept of a 'Higher Power', but I slid over that and did my best to work the programme. After a year or so, I learned to take responsibility for my behaviour, and I tried to make amends with all of the people I had hurt when manic. I wrote letters of apology to the lamas at KTD and to Trungpa Rinpoche.

After two years in AA, I went off the deep end again. I got wildly manic and drank a fifth (of a gallon) of bourbon, thereby burning all of my bridges with my AA sponsor and other AA friends. After witnessing my sponsor's failure to understand the difference between a manic episode and a bender, I could no longer go back to AA. Instead, I wound up with the first of many commitments to the state hospital in Augusta. What I had learned in AA opened my eyes to the value of peer support, and I took solace in talking with fellow patients, in giving and receiving peer support. With the positive energy of mania, I had learned how to cheer people up and give them hope. In this way I directed the energy that had been so destructive to a constructive purpose.

The practice of compassion

When I got home I wrote a letter of apology to my AA sponsor. Making amends was a discipline that I learned in AA and took to heart, along with peer support. It was the first time I took responsibility for the way I had behaved and damaged others when I was manic.

I made up my mind to live alone and find some way to carry out Khenpo Rinpoche's instructions. At the hospital, when my psychologist had asked me what my support system would be, I did not even know what he was talking about. I had become used to living with no family, no friends and not even a therapist. The woman I lived with for a while, my former AA cronies and most of my family, who lived far away, had pretty much given up on me.

When I left the hospital, I heard of a new organization in Portland – the Alliance for the Mentally Ill (AMI). I joined, even though the members were mostly families, not mental health consumers. Immediately I sought out my peers – the sons and daughters of AMI members – and joined their small support group, called Consumer Coalition for the Mentally Ill. Before too long I became the leader of the group, and we grew from a handful of members to a non-profit organization that supported mental health consumers. To reflect our newly radical stance, we renamed ourselves the Portland Coalition for the Psychiatrically Labeled. It was a joyful time for me. I prolifically produced sing-along and poetry groups, a slide show, a poetry book, peer support groups and even political demonstrations. I introduced advocacy for clients in the mental health system in Maine, and wrote successful grants to give us funding for an office and for our advocacy and peer support work. I followed my instincts in advocating locally and around the state, a little astonished to find that, for the first time in my life, I could play a useful and important role. I thought back in gratitude to Rinpoche's advice to work with other people in the community, certain that this was exactly what he had in mind.

In developing the Coalition, I experienced what was later to be called the 'helper principle' by researchers. The idea is that when a person who is wounded works to help others who are similarly wounded, both benefit. I had received a taste of this in AA, where I found peers helping peers and working for their mutual recovery. I began to appreciate the Buddhist emphasis on compassion as the active side of enlightenment. I understood that merely following a regimen of prayer would not have been enough for me – it might result in only the abstract wisdom of faith without a ground in reality. I had to learn to truly care about others. So I worked to accomplish for mental health consumers in Maine what at that time (in 1981) had been achieved in few other places – a peer-run organization that believed in empowerment and respect. I even managed to sneak in a little Dharma through the Coalition's motto, a standard Buddhist maxim: 'To help ourselves and others'. I was in my forties, and those were the best days of my life.

But this was still only half good enough. Even with all of the gratification from my work, I still had to deal with fiery psychotic episodes that damaged both myself and others. At least once every year I succumbed to the seduction of mania, and tried in desperation to recapture luminosity and find the 'ultimate' meaning of the universe. Each of these episodes ended in a crash of bleak depression, and during one of these I tried to commit suicide. This pattern went on for seven years. In between times, I tried to be both a good Dharma practitioner and a faithful Christian. I sang in the choir at St Peter's. I joined a Buddhist study group that met weekly and dutifully sat with them for hours at a time, even though I knew that this unstructured practice was dangerous for me and raised manic energy. I had not returned to KTD since the fire alarm incident, afraid that the lamas would reject me.

But the magical successes with the Coalition ceased and soured. The board of directors would no longer tolerate my frequent relapses. Worse, some of these persons, along with the staff, became heady with the power and influence that the director and I had earned through hard work, and they wanted this power for themselves. Several of them worked actively to subvert the administration, and they succeeded.

I was devastated. I felt as if I had returned to square one – once again a total failure. I was bewildered that a project started with such good advice from my teacher, and carried out with such joy and success, could just as quickly turn to dust in my hands. I could only conclude that my fault had been in not learning to control my manic episodes, and I chose to follow the Buddhist maxim to 'take the blame upon yourself'. I had to acknowledge the Dharma teaching, emphasized over and over again, that everything without exception is impermanent. I wrote a letter to Khenpo Rinpoche explaining that I had followed his advice, and describing what had happened. I asked whether it would be possible for me to return to KTD for further study and meditation instruction.

The discipline of practice

Much to my surprise, rather than regarding me as a *persona non grata*, Rinpoche chided me for not keeping in touch with him and said that I would be welcome to come back to KTD. I immediately visited there and went several times over the next year. I resolved to move permanently to the monastery and perhaps to carry out my original intention of living the rest of my life in retreat and prayer. I carried out my decision in steps, however, wanting to act from wisdom rather than impulse.

In my first interviews with Rinpoche, I requested that he give me a meditation practice that I could do at home, but that would not exacerbate my manic energies. Rinpoche explained that a regular discipline was more important than the length of time practised. He instructed me to sit two times a day for only ten minutes each, and to start this practice with a few repetitions of the well-known Tibetan mantra, *om mani padme hum*. He gave me a picture of a Kagyu lineage master to put on a shrine, along with six little bronze bowls to fill with water and a string of beads, called a *mala*, to count repetitions of the mantra. When I followed these instructions at home, I felt at last a confidence in practice and a stability of mind that I had not before been able to achieve.

On my last visit to KTD before moving to Woodstock, I requested Rinpoche to give me the empowerment for the Green Tara puja, the public meditation observed every day at 5am. Green Tara is the female deity sometimes called the 'mother of the buddhas', who is most revered by Tibetan practitioners. She represents at the same time motherly love and profound wisdom, and is often called 'Drolma', or Lady. I always felt drawn to Tara practice, even though it was so difficult and demanding that few of the American residents at KTD made it to the early morning prayers, preferring to attend the other ceremonies offered later in the day.

Rinpoche agreed to give me the *lung* empowerment, which would consist of his reciting the text and giving me a blessing. I came to his room equipped with the traditional white scarf and an offering. I put the scarf around his neck and gave him the envelope with my offering, and he returned the scarf and put it around my neck. Then we talked for a few moments. He repeated how pleased he was with the work I had done for the Portland Coalition. He said that I had helped a lot of people, and this made him very happy. He also approved my success in following the meditations that he had given me earlier. We began the empowerment by reciting a few traditional prayers, including the refuge prayer. Then Rinpoche held on his lap a copy of the Green Tara puja and, holding it, recited by memory the chant of '21 Praises', which is the heart of the practice. When doing the puja, one repeats these 21 Praises, first two times, then three times, and finally seven times. In general, the 21 Praises extol all the varied qualities of Tara, praising both her wisdom and her compassionate action. When he had finished, Rinpoche touched the top of my head with the manuscript and gave it to me. He then bumped the top of my head with his head, a traditional Tibetan gesture of affection.

I practised the Green Tara sadhana at home so that by the time I finally arrived in Woodstock I knew a little bit more about what I was doing. After I arrived, I rented an apartment in town, as I still did not feel comfortable with the secular residents at KTD. Now that I had finally received empowerment to perform a major practice, I felt less inclined to renounce everything else. I had never really wanted to be a nun. In any case, for over a year I arose before dawn and drove up the mountain in pitch blackness to practise Green Tara with two or three other students, led by Bardor Tulku Rinpoche. I found this deeply moving, and because the energies aroused by sadhana are carefully channelled, every day my mental stability increased. The structure of the practice, and the physical elements of it – chanting, hand gestures, movements with the bell and dorje and the gifts of torma at the end – all had a grounding effect that brought the wisdom aspect of prayer together with the action aspect of compassion. In Vajrayana Buddhism, it is believed that performing tantric practices can bring about transformations in one's mind and body – not anything new and different, but a rechannelling of conflicting emotions and other imperfections to healthy and enlightened versions of the same energies. That, of course, was what I was looking for. All of these years I had looked for a way to achieve recovery from the manic episodes that had disrupted my life so badly.

As I continued my daily prayers, I began to notice changes in my behaviour. My thinking did not change and my beliefs remained the same. But I began to notice that, when I became deeply involved in practice, particularly the 21 Praises, something happened in my brain and body that could be described as a 'rewiring'. This might be explained as a movement of the 'winds', or spiritual energies, or simply as a rerouting of habitual pathways in the nervous system. In any case, although I did not feel fundamentally different in any way, I noticed that other people reacted to me differently – I seemed to be less of a threat to them, and to inspire trust in others. My mind was more stable and serene, and less crowded with anxious thoughts. I noticed that I had remained free from psychosis for two full years, including the year that I had practised at home. This was twice as long as I had ever remained stable before.

Encouraged at this improvement, I began to look for volunteer work in the Woodstock community. At first I worked for a warm line (helpline) in town. Then I discovered that there was a small peer support group for mental health consumers in Poughkeepsie, the location of the state hospital where I was incarcerated several years before. I joined the group and became one of its leaders. Once again, we formed a non-profit organization that became a model for other groups around the state. When we opened our first office and drop-in centre, Khenpo Rinpoche came and conferred a blessing on our new facilities. He again told me how pleased he was that I was doing this work.

Soon I was no longer able to keep up my early morning drives to KTD. But I did continue my Green Tara practice, doing it at home for an hour and a half each morning. It stood me in good stead. I found that, even while doing the very public and stressful work of our consumer-run group, I managed to relate to other people with a calm and equanimity that I had not been able to muster with the Coalition. I continued in this work for another four years, until the New York group also fell prey to infighting and power struggles, and I left to take a job as therapist with a Buddhist-based mental health programme in another state. At that point, I had been free of manic episodes for over six years.

Discipline resumed

Ironically, the Buddhist treatment programme turned out to be a disappointment, for I found myself in the same kind of conflict with people there as I had experienced at Karma Chöling and with my study group in Maine. As a 'provider' myself, I felt alienated from the peer advocacy that had been rewarding in the past, and I let my Dharma practice slide. I could no longer bring myself to chant all of the Tibetan words that now seemed alien to me.

Not surprisingly, within a couple of years my mind took off for 'parts unknown', and I endured another manic episode that resulted in eviction from my apartment and another hospitalization. Resigning from my job, I moved to Florida, where I had some consulting work, and where I had a connection with yet another drop-in centre in Fort Lauderdale. I chose to live in rural Florida, in a quiet apartment overlooking a lake. I still did not resume my Dharma practice, not really knowing how to get back to it, but I found that living in peace and solitude was an important component to maintaining my mental stability. I also resumed taking lithium, which I had cut off just before the manic episode. I began doing some work for the South Florida drop-in centre, while still living in my retreat in the country. All went well for nearly five years, and I maintained my sanity. Then, all of a sudden, the drop-in centre seemed to implode with employee conflicts, pursuits of power and mean-spiritedness. I lost my job and once again it seemed that everything I had worked for over the years had crumbled.

I realized that it was time to go back to KTD and take a refresher course in Dharma practice. Embarrassed that I had been away so long, I tentatively arranged for a week-long visit. I was apprehensive as I drove to Woodstock from the airport, but once I reached KTD, I felt as if I were home again. Nothing had changed. When I talked with Rinpoche, I found that even he was the same! He was somewhat heavier than before, but looked to be in excellent health. I was the one who had changed, for I was much older now, nearly 60, and suffering from osteoarthritis, a handicap I did not have before. I was greeted graciously by the KTD residents, many of whom had been there years ago, and who remembered events as if they occurred only yesterday. Best of all, they treated me with the respect given to a senior practitioner.

I explained to Rinpoche what had happened with my work as a peer advocate, and I confessed the difficulty I had in getting back to practice. As always, he was sympathetic and kind, and he instructed me in prayers that were less demanding than the hour-and-a-half-long sadhana I had done before. Before I returned to Florida, he gave me a gift that would help me with my practice and remind me of him and my friends at KTD. It is a silver amulet on a red cord that I now wear every day.

Back in my peaceful and solitary home, I continue to do my new practice. Even though it is not as strenuous as the long Green Tara I did before, it has, as before, helped me to stabilize my mind and to present myself to others in a way that is beneficial. Although I do not feel particularly wise or holy – or even-tempered, for that matter – my friends and co-workers often tell me that they admire my calm and serenity. This amazes me, but I take it as the best way to gauge whether my practice is working. As long as I can be helpful to other people and maintain my own wellbeing, I will be satisfied. I have now been free of psychosis for over 15 years, with the one exception of the episode in Massachusetts. I hope that at long last I have lived up to the implications of my refuge name, Karma Tsultrim Zangmo. After all, 'discipline' is my middle name, and it is through the discipline of daily practice that I found safety and wellbeing. Through helping other people I found a way to see the basic goodness in both myself and others.

Chapter 10

Grace

Cathy Conroy

Cathy Conroy is a former mental health advocate from Goulburn, Australia. Presently she is teaching kindergarten and 11- and 12-year-old children, after 24 years away from the classroom.

> I am interested in the retention of ties and friendships with mental health consumers. In particular, the plight of the mentally ill remains utmost in my mind, since I am always sharing with them something of the same journey. A great spirit of care exists in the community and it is my strong recognition that the Holy Spirit is truly among us.

Grace – an overview

On the underground platform in my mind's eye I saw in the dark tunnel many memories light up. I saw spirituality and mental health in the cave of the heart alight together.

This journey is the description of one passenger endeavouring to make sense of the encounter with spirituality and a bipolar state. It is the discovery too, along the way, of the light of transcendence – the Holy Spirit.

> For it is by God's grace that you have been saved through faith. It is not the result of your own efforts, but God's gift, so that no one can boast about it. God has made us what we are, and in our union with Christ Jesus he has created us for a life of good deeds, which he has already prepared for us to do.
>
> Ephesians (2: 9–10)

Grace

The Holy Spirit comes when we are receptive. He does not compel. He approaches so meekly that we may not even notice. If we would know the Holy Spirit, we need to examine ourselves in the light of the Gospel teaching, to detect any other presence, which may prevent the Holy Spirit from entering into our souls. We must not wait for God to force himself on us without our consent. God respects and does not constrain us. It is amazing how God humbles himself before us. He loves us with a tender love, not haughtily, not with condescension. And when we open our hearts to him we are overwhelmed by the conviction that he is indeed our Father. The soul then worships with love.

Sophrony (2002)

Make certain, then, that the light in you is not darkness. If your whole body is full of light, with no part of it in darkness it will be bright all over, as when a lamp shines on you with its brightness.

Luke (11: 33–36)

The juxtaposed states of light and dark play on the soul, longing for resolutions of deep inner conflict. All the allied forces gather together in their varying dimensions, awaiting the spiritual stamina for reconciliation that comes from an infusion of grace and the natural suspension of psychotic activity, which so disturbs the mind, body and spirit. The raw nerves of fear in this state of fragility are exposed. The recognition of the rising struggle between good and evil becomes apparent, and yet the Holy Spirit – at the very core of the soul – defends and protects while the eruptions are painful and frightening.

This can be such a terrifying and baffling journey, but the 'fire and ice', the light and the dark, are transforming the very soul whose journey into eternity has well and truly begun.

The stunning contrast between the events of a night and a day is one of the most vivid recollections flooding my mind and my heart inexorably.

Day: It was Easter and in memory of the Lord, my husband, my parents-in-law and I broke bread and shared some red wine around a small, yellow Formica table. At this time, in 1978, in our tiny farm cottage, 'Pine Lodge', just outside Goulburn, NSW, in a heightened state, I listened to *Panis Angelicus* and felt deeply grateful for our simple rented home. My interior was, however, safely held from view.

Night: Enfolded in the night, yet wide awake, I was taken, in reality, in mind, body and spirit to Our Lord as He trudged to Calvary. The journey was arduous, intense in the extreme, all encompassing, and a total emptying and draining was experienced throughout the night as my whole person responded to this place of oneness.

As the hours went by and I remained in exhausted darkness and union, an indelible impression of supreme mystery was cast on my heart and mind. It was a 'cloud of unknowing'. The experience, overwhelmingly, was one of being within the very depths of my spirit, and conscious to me.

From a state of wrenching exhaustion, the early morning light arrived and instantaneously energy and strength flowed throughout my whole body. Since I knew nothing of an event such as this, I kept all to myself, for there was a deep intuition of unnamed spiritual experience that I needed to keep locked away at this time. I was overawed and taken totally from my moorings. It was many years ago but I recall the dark and light clearly.

In the new day I stood with my mother-in-law in the warm rays of the sun, replenished. I fell silent ... 'We love because God first loved us' (1 John, 4: 19).

The nature of disorder

Bipolar disorder is a serious mental illness. The insidious nature of this illness cannot be underestimated. It can start off fairly innocuously and grow to proportions that can be difficult to contain.

The disorder takes somewhat of a defined course and can be related to changes in the season. Losing sleep can activate an episode.

Spun out and desperately weary from the heightened states and the sometimes incumbent psychosis, the person with the bipolar disorder attempts valiantly to continue working, striving and achieving – close to being broken, ashamed, stripped and burnt out. At this point the spiritual side is hardly identified and a battery of medication is supplied to dampen the mood swings. The spiritual aspects of the episode often remain essentially undisclosed. In all fragmented thinking, even at times when there is disorientation, there is a search for some kind of order, which could well be recognized as a signpost for deeper reality, for a more truthful insight. Discarded, however, as irrational thought, valuable understanding is often lost.

When depression strikes, the person slinks into another pattern, unable to communicate effectively or to meet the normal demands of existence. This is tremendously shattering for the individual and the family and friends of the affected person. From a point of utopia comes a sharp diminishment.

Throughout recent history we have numerous examples of famous men and women who have had this dreaded illness. Many of these people were/are highly creative musicians, poets, writers and philosophers. In fact there are such a large number of brilliant people suffering from this illness, one must ask oneself why this is so.

The way I see it is that the barrage of events in the mind and emotions somehow finely tunes creative spirits. The thoughts and feelings are somewhat deeper, but the precipice is not always in front. As a consequence, the higher the manic depressive climbs (in a mind sense), the lower the drop, iced and hell-bent, so to speak.

GM Hopkins (Gardener, 1953) reveals the height and depth of his own such experience:

No worst, there is none pitched past pitch of grief
More pangs will, schooled at forepangs, wilder wring ...
O the mind, has mountains; cliffs of fall,
Frightful, sheer, no-man fathomed.

And then he expresses the beauty of the story of rising. In *Hurrahing in Harvest*, Hopkins exclaims:

I walk, I lift up, I lift up heart, eyes,
Down all that glory in the heavens to glean our Saviour;
And, eyes, heart, what looks, what lips yet gave you a Rapturous love's
Greeting of realer, of rounder replies? ...

Climbing out of torment

It was in my twenties that psychiatrists confirmed I had a bipolar disorder and I have been treated for that ever since. A profound religious conversion in September 1998 on top of a strong spiritual sense has contributed to a new and different understanding of mental health and spirituality. At that time I wrote with a sense of great certainty:

Give thanks to the Lord, tell His name. Make known His deeds among the peoples. Oh sing to Him! Sing His praise! Tell all his wonderful works!

(Psalm 104)

I am going to give her back her vineyards and make the valley of Achor a gateway of hope.

(Hosea 2: 15)

I am summonsed to appear before the Most High.

Robed in embroidered silk garments and hair knotted with plaited strands of gold ...

A thousand million sparks of joy explode – deep longing for metanoia.
Flooding tears, great fear, vibrations of hope for my heart to shatter open;

Transform my dull mind through the blazing fire of your love and alleviate
the internal riot of my faithlessness and doubt.

Illuminate the ebb and flow in my consciousness,

Your love that I am so slow to identify.

Could you work within me Lord, sustaining such longings and feelings?

You have forgiven me, Majesty – Lord and yet I weep and shake and have
sadness covering me.

                                                                            C Conroy

Lure me lead me out of the wilderness and speak to my heart.

                                                                        (Hosea 2: 15)

And so it was that I attended the St Peter and Paul's Goulburn parish mission. At that time my mental illness had become more savage, creating terrible strains in the family. My mother, who heart-brokenly listened to my sobbing despair, reached out with deep love, on a daily basis.

I felt not only the full array of manic depressive symptoms, but a head cluttered with racing thoughts, intense anger and a wild and shocking inability to see worth in myself; a desire, too, to denigrate the people I loved. I was a terrible mess and I wondered how I would ever escape the chaos.

I wrote to Our Lord at this time, apologizing for my constant longing for reassurance. I asked if I had betrayed the light of Him in me, beseeching a sign of strength. I cried out:

Take me in your arms universe of glory,
Your emerald afternoon of dancing light.
Your new season of elm leaves shining.
Cover this sinking sadness.
Cradle this woman of sorrows, of weeping, of torn heart; bereft, forlorn.
Why do I go there again and again, Lord, stripped and lost of life?

At this time I was working as a mental health consumer advocate. I was observing my role but there was within me a level of disintegration. I had been hiding the anguished levels of my mind and heart and it was becoming more difficult to do the job properly in such circumstances. My memory and my whole physical state were badly affected. My heart was tormented by rapid cycling mood swings. The sinister envy I held for those that could work well, who were 'normal', was terribly painful.

Deep compassion for the mentally ill remained, but the fragility of my mind meant much ineffectualness. Trudging up the cliff, with a colossal millstone around my neck, was defeating the hope of ever achieving anything. Yet in the days with mentally ill people there was the recognition of a sense of joy, some shared creativity and the connection with extremities of sadness, depression, frustration and delusion. Most important, however, were the strong bonds of trust, friendship and love.

Very often my perspective of mental health was seen differently to that of the clinicians and psychiatrists. The executive summary report from the Surgeon General of the US Public Health Service (1999) stated that mental health is:

> ... the successful performance of mental function, resulting in productive activities, fulfilling relationship with other people, and the ability to adapt to change and to cope with adversity; from early childhood until late life, mental health is the springboard of thinking and communication skills, learning, emotional growth, resilience and self-esteem.

To my mind it is much more than this; the recognition of God's abiding grace in our lives, primarily leading us, is paramount. 'We can say that grace is the spirit lovingly at work in our lives, empowering our best efforts' (Groome, 2002).

In a very special book, *Healing*, Father Richard McAlear, OMI (1999), stated:

> Many illnesses, physical and emotional, are rooted in the spiritual – especially the inability to accept forgiveness and receive pardon and peace.

He spoke of 'Jesus' compassion and forgiveness as the fundamental healing gift'. To embrace this gift is the basic experience of deliverance – freedom from guilt, recrimination, self-punishment and condemnation.

Freedman et al. (1975) define psychosis as a:

> Mental disorder in which a person's mental capacity, affective response, and capacity to recognise reality, to communicate, and to relate to others are impaired enough to interfere with his capacity to deal with the ordinary demands of life.

There remains in the psychosis, however, threads of meaning that can be woven into the fabric along the way. Moreover, the continuing recollection of the mental and emotional events contained in the psychosis seem to express something of a deeper yearning: a longing to understand the heart and mind – however disordered. The growing consciousness of the effects of the redemption of the Lord's body and blood, within, transforms us. Shafts of light shine in the darkness inspiring faith and hope.

In *The Hound of Heaven*, Francis Thompson (1960) expresses the way in which he ran from the Lord:

> I fled Him, down the nights and down the days:
> I fled Him, down the arches of the years;

I fled Him, down the labyrinthine ways
of my own mind: and in the midst of tears
I hid from Him, and under running laughter
Up vistaed hopes I sped;
And shot precipitated ...

There comes a place of real kindling of Christ's Holy Spirit. The real presence is believed in, and the mysterious, gracious and overwhelming
knowledge of Our Lord's love is embraced.

The journey of recovery

The true sense of recovery is something of the same journey for us all,
although we walk different paths, swim different seas. In the long run we
seek the same destination of love. A growing respect and faith in the individual narrative of the mentally ill is vitally important. The reality and
sense of personal integrity is a deepening movement. Awakening to the
world on a sacred journey more intense and unified is indeed a path of
grace, new discovery, meaning, responsibility and direction.

I had swept my energies alarmingly close to those for whom I advocated and had become vulnerable, perhaps more so than ever. However, the
values of empathy and compassion in the long haul remained of committed importance. The mentally ill person is often stripped of much
personal belief, identity and self-worth, and the reality of psychotic events
can become a construct of truth, an embedded neural tune. Helping to
change the story at the right vantage point, with the very integrity of the
person deeply respected, is critical, and at times I found myself out of my
depth. I needed to come to the understanding of just letting change happen without any of my imperatives.

Now comes a time of deep reflection. It is only from a distance that a
truer knowledge of events, deemed to be solely psychotic, can be viewed
as part of the path to God. 'No human being comes into the presence of
the all-holy God without passing through the fire of purification'
(Johnston, 1995). For a long time I had been trying to understand what
was psychotic and what was spiritual; it became evident that the spirit was
deeply entwined in the psyche, in fact the whole being.

The heightened state of mania and devastating depression, where lack
of control and chaos prevail, is truly different from the experience of the
flight of the spirit, which leaves a deeper sense of prayerfulness, mystery
and vision in its wake and heralds the strong voice: 'Let us open our eyes
and ears and our hearts, it is Christ the Lord, it is He.' Healing for me has
been the gift of clarity in the sacraments of the Blessed Eucharist,
Reconciliation and the Anointing of the Sick. These sacraments provide

great strength and protection in the times of angst, terror and confusion. This is the time where the 'dark side of the personality flows into the conscious mind and is brought to light' (Johnston, 1995). Yet, it is not only in darkness that healing comes; it is also present in all shades of light. As the dying Yoganada prayed: 'In this your temple with your own hand light the lamp of your love, turn my darkness into light. Turn my darkness into light.'

Optimism

Optimistic that more of the labyrinth could be known through love and friendship meant a constant drawing into greater consciousness, as the conflict of sorrow and joy created a catalyst for personal change. Important embers of reality take much time to ignite in the journey of recovery. Trust in the initial experience of the mentally ill, and instilling a virtue-based claim at the magistrate hearing or in the tribunal, filled the sensitive mentally ill person with words of acceptance and encouragement. This is a place where one requires a sense of support and knowledge of intrinsic goodness. This will be needed for the times down the path when the experience of loss of personal belief is likely. The abiding responsibility was to stay strong, to joke, to rejoice and to be happy so that the sunshine could be forever spread around; and to lift those not so well off into the same stream of optimism and strength.

Although God had been putting so many things in place for me, it seemed that the St Peter and Paul mission was an answer to my new cry in the wilderness. My initial aspiration was how wonderful it would be if God relieved the sometimes crushing mental blow just a little. After all, in every psychosis – in every mental break of dark depression and unbridled leaping manic gallop – the Lord had spoken to me so many times through music, in prayer and in family love. Not unusual for the mentally ill. Mystical paths so secret and ineffable are carved from the demolition of fear and chaos, with the acceptance of forgiveness.

Patience

My hope of being healed *immediately* of my mental illness by the Holy Spirit did not happen in the way I anticipated. However, a new clarity and healing led me to understand the way in which my mental health and spirituality are irrevocably linked. The slow movement towards authentic thought and action is perfected through the grace, mercy and goodness of God.

Every person is acceptable to God. We are created in his image and therefore we are valued and loved. Each is loved into life, beyond sin, failure and disappointment. Today matters more than yesterday. Wholeness flows from the humble acceptance of love despite unworthiness: it understands mercy: it accepts grace.

McAlear (1999)

In *No Boundary*, Ken Wilber (1985) wrote:

At the bottom of your soul, is the soul of humanity itself and a divine, transcendent soul, leading from bondage to liberation, from enchantment to awakening, from time to eternity from death to immortality.

In this was the beginning of an appreciation of the depth and essence of every person, and the way in which the individual journey is studded with lights and darkness and kaleidoscopic views patterning and repatterning, developing and evolving as the intimacy with the divine enters more intensely and transforms. Interestingly, Nelson Mandela in his inaugural speech in 1994 said: 'It is our light, not our darkness, that most frightens us.' Meister Eckhart described darkness in this way:

What is this darkness? What is its name? Call it an aptitude for sensitivity. Call it a rich sensitivity, which will make you whole. Call it your potential vulnerability.

Journeying through the layers of consciousness leads to the kind of hope that Emily Dickinson (Browning et al., 1993) spoke of:

Hope is a thing with feathers
That perches in the soul
And sings the tune without the words
And never stops at all.

St John of the Cross said:

In The Dark Night, one must be content with a loving and peaceful attentiveness to God, and live without the concern, without the effort and without the desire to taste or feel Him.

And yet, without bidding, when the trees were laden with wattle and a gentle mist sprinkled Goulburn town, contrasting shades of bright light and dark sparked new search.

The eventide pathos swells and falls
and the shadows lengthen.
Now to the west the glowing embers of
the day burst brightly and are gently hushed.
My heart whimpering still, after solitary confinement

pleads for forgiveness and freedom.
Ocean of balm's love assuage and deluge me
Renewing hope, reconciling with joy ...
Breath of the spirit, Father of love,
the life of the Son,
sound the harmonies of peace.

                                                                    C Conroy

Oh sing my soul, my saviour God to Thee.
How Great Thou Art.
How Great Thou Art.

The word *'metanoia'* had a ring to it for me and, in my superficiality, hope of a *change of heart* was to be simply like a dark night merging into a bright new day, although not quite so smoothly. *Metanoia* is the biblical word for conversion and this is how it is defined by a Redemptorist priest, Father Kevin O'Shea (1971), in *On Trial for Hope*, he said:

> Suppose someone blindfolds you, then twists and twirls you round and round until you get dizzy and you don't know where you are. Your hands move out in search of something you can touch, something that will give you a bearing, a sense of direction. You find something; and you find some-thing else; and slowly you begin to feel where you are again, and to take a few steps in a new direction. That, in a human way, is the experience of metanoia. It is like learning to walk again when you are lost, when you have no securities.

Pope Paul VI described *metanoia* as 'a change of heart that is an intimate, total change and renewal of the entire man, of all his opinions, judge-ments, and decisions, which takes place in him in the light of the holiness and kindness of God, shown to him and given to him in Jesus Christ'.

> How wonderfully is man's love transformed by the interior experience of this nothingness and this nowhere ... He who patiently abides in this dark-ness will be comforted and feel again a confidence about this destiny, for gradually he will see his past sins healed by grace. The pain continues yet he knows it will end, for even now it grows less intense. Slowly he begins to realise that the suffering he endures is not hell at all but his purgatory.

                                          (From *Cloud of Unknowing*, Anon, 1973)

An experience I had, one day before Lent in 1999, spoke to me lovingly and tenderly:

Come to the time of the harvest as mortal flesh falls away in the sun;

The Holy Spirit is now and inebriates my mind

Renewing and transforming my mortality with infusions of sacred spirit in blood and bone.

Sparkling poplars flash and dance with lightning flickerings, silvered streaming in the sun; and I in elevated thought slow become sober – nothing to exchange, lost and without measure and in exquisite unknown,

O Holy Spirit creation come ...

C Conroy

This fleeting, but illuminating, experience of oneness intimated and beckoned, and was felt unexpectedly in a cloudburst of joy. Could this be mysterious gracing transcendence, *a gift*, leaving enlightenment and love and new explorations of greater interiority?

There is a sense of certainty that full commitment to my faith has enhanced the ongoing healing of my mind and heart. As one is taken to a greater depth, spiritually, a deeper appreciation of the Other arises. It had become apparent that my imagination focused on self, somehow creating the speed and Icarus-type experiences that in time gave way to falls and psychosis. And yet out of the morass, the sense of being 'held' and 'holding on' prevailed.

Our right and loving relationship with God must permeate with other relationships – with self, others, and creation. The measure of Christian spirituality will always be the life-giving quality of our relationships.

Groome (2002)

One day at mass, a profound and intense inner experience occurred in the tiny Goulburn Base Hospital Chapel. I tried to encapsulate something of the experience, to put into words the state of my thoughts and feelings and my need to express my perception at that time.

Holy Spirit in the Temple and in the Heart

Quickly and silently the case of my heart was opened;
a burning mass, this forge cried for the Lord of Hosts
and in the longing, tears of joy and sorrow swept through my heart being
   renewed.
I concealed the tumult, the magnificent, indescribable mystery, I wondered
   if I should ever be able to share these life transforming events.
I thank you Holy Lord wondrous of the whole firmament only Lord and
   king.
Abide with me.

Lush red velvet rose
blood petals endearing
ready to receive the Host of the Lord
what could I say, how could I say it
Rapturous space, rapturous love
tenuous music, Holy Lord. Thirst of desire.

In the becoming of the being,
the making of the made,
the descent of the Holy Spirit of CREATION,
comes the knowledge of the knower,
sees the agape of the Divine, the charge of all beings.

Iced, foggy morning
Ring of temple fire
Mt Horeb day
Lightning struck being
subside gently now
fall back to nothing
Nada te turbe ...
Oh my God.

The music fills the air
sweetest nostalgia rising
kettles in the wake
Hold still for the Lord's sake.

Gather the fragile fire and ice,
put it in your basket of Love,
blend it into moonshine,
send it above in hope.
Tongue of Fire.

Elected Silence.

Ruffled red feathers of redbreast
echo the Agnus Dei of Easter Joy.
Arising now, creations feast, creations delight.
The blood of the lamb
is the blood of forgiveness
The blood of the lamb ... the unity of all.
SHOUT, DANCE, SING.

For He has Risen indeed Alleluia
the marvels of the Lord, OH.
STAY VERY STILL ...
RISING HEART
PEARL of GREAT PRICE. AMOUR!

Un-tie my hands, unbind my ankles
Beam your light into the window of my soul
Bring your solace to the dispossessed refugees of mental disease
You know I will serve if I may,
Take me on, as you serve me.
Since you are mine and thee are theirs
And here the eternal harmonic of light and sound
Streams with your glory and your hope.

C Conroy

Converging paths

The mental health path and the spiritual path are converging roads in the clearing and in the forest. However, they traverse territory so different for us all, despite containing synchronous motifs. Thoughts that were once hushed and cloistered jettison, when the imagination is allowed to freely roam. On some occasions we wish we had not ventured so far unaccompanied. 'Oh Shenandoah, it's far I wander ...'

The inner territory of the person with a bipolar disorder contains great capacity for rebirth and growth.

A clean heart create for me, O God
and a steadfast spirit renew within me.
Cast me not out from your presence,
and your holy spirit take not from me.

(Psalm 51: 12–13)

The valleys of the cyclical states, the mountainous terrains and the tossing winds create a longing to be led to 'restful pastures'. Painful psychosis – the dark in the light of the soul's journey – is, in a sense, a sharing in the cross of Christ, perceived in spiritual recollection and experience. Acceptance of my born identity allows the light of Christ to shine, to enliven my life in my relationships with others and to know Christ's presence in my heart, within my whole being.

Tutored by mood swings, the capricious spirit becomes partially prepared for deep joy and sorrow. Direct experience of the spiritual dimension is immediate, hard to define and deeply touching. The Holy Spirit gradually enlightening the heart and mind fills the cavities and the cracks of psychotic thought and activity, gluing it with 'the lava of love', the very love of the Lord himself.

At the time of the Russian submarine disaster, the spirit flew to the deepest level of my psyche. It was a precipitously low place and I felt so afraid. The feelings I had led to a psychosis and I just could not cope. Fear, combining with lack of understanding, as the valley of darkness and

I remained there, lost, alone and in terror, until rescued and taken to higher ground. This appeared to be a metaphor for the plight of the submariners. The holy oil on my hands and forehead miraculously burnt when I received the sacrament of the Anointing of the Sick.

On the feast on the Ascension in 2000 I expressed the experience of this time:

> Immanent and transcendent Lord of the universe,
> Holding together all hands; offering forth
> A glory unknown, ever felt.
> A scale unimpinged, Oh Lord, Oh God
> You are beautiful ... unimagined words ...
> Visions unnavigated; synergistic dance of all peoples.
> Please take my two hands if you would my Lord Jesus Christ
> Here they are so little, wiping away ecstatic tears,
> in the flowing river of your glorious love.
> Thank you Holy Spirit for joyful revelations.
> Thank you sweet Eucharistic perfection.
> This day.

The flight of the spirit was extraordinary. It shot forth seemingly with the speed of light and then ground into the ocean depths. The spirit charged through me and I was excited sometimes and terrified at others, hardly knowing what to feel. The climax of events flashed instantaneously with the soaring and plunging.

Running one day in the park, listening to Handel's Messiah, the utmost certainty of the words, 'And in my flesh I shall see God ...' struck me through and through. I pinched myself as I felt a heightened sense beyond any words.

> (You) will have the strength to grasp the breadth and length, the height and depth, until knowing the love of Christ, which is beyond all knowledge, you are filled with the utter fullness of God.

> (Eph. 3: 16–18)

It was St Patrick's day, a joyous day, and of the Redeemer I wrote:

Hail Redeemer
Shooting into all the tomorrows of eternity
And falling fast through eternity
The tiny fragment of today, yesterday and tomorrow
is untold surprise;

This abyss of melancholy holds the death of Our Lord
and this ecstasy proclaims His resurrection
Holding fast to His rebirth,
As fast as I hold onto mine, through Him
is the realisation of fire and ice
coming together in time.

C Conroy.

Teilhard de Chardin, whose thought and feeling encompasses the massive range of the human condition, said illuminatedly:

In truth, each of us is called upon to respond, by a pure and incommunicable harmonic, to the universal note. When through the progress of our hearts towards love of the whole, we feel, stretching out above our various strivings and desires, the exuberant simplicity of an impulse in which all remain distinct, it is then that at the heart of the mass of human energy we each draw nearer to the fullness of our effective powers of our personality.

When the knowledge of the buttressing force of the Divine within and without is deeply acknowledged as supreme mystery, fortifying love and grace floods our souls and holds an intense hope for love, freedom and peace for us all. It is too, the recognition of the wealth and dynamism of the person's bipolar states harnessed in this way, that creative endeavour is recognized as gift. Plotinus (quoted in O'Brien, 1964) says:

We must close our eyes
and invoke a new manner of seeing
and wakefulness that is the birthright of us all.

Sri Aurobindo defined the seasons of the heart in this way:

In spring: The hushed heart hears the unuttered word.

In summer: Become and live the knowledge thou hast; then is thy knowledge the living God within thee.

In autumn: A divine force shall flow through tissue and cell and take the charge of breath and speech and act.

In winter: Pain is the hand of nature sculpturing us to greatness.

Knowledge of heart and mind

Mental health and spirituality is about mind and heart knowledge – becoming awake to the life within. And it is here that we are talking about bridges: new bridges, the bridges between mental health and spirituality, between light and darkness, between the self and the soul, between insight and revelation. Spirituality is not just one aspect of mental health: spirituality is the very core. It is the seen and the unseen.

Spirit of Renewal, quieten our anxieties and arouse our confidence.
Ocean waves splash over our sadness.
Salty waters bathe the wounds of all those with mental illness.
Unite us with each other in our impassioned quest for love and hope, gratitude and grace.
Searching beyond horizons
and past long cast shadows
dreaming ocean salt spray, depths unfathomed
beholding string clouds, whisking spun moondust
still unquenched thirst of you (darling) charged mystery
rocked, swathed rolling in awesome might, Maker.

Conroy (1999)

References

Anon (1973) Cloud of Unknowing. New York: Doubleday, Image Books.

Browning EB, Dickinson E and Rosetti C (1993) A Voice Within Three Women Poets. London: Aurum Press.

Conroy C (1999) Fire and Ice. In: Barker P, Campbell P and Davidson B (eds) From the Ashes of Experience: reflections on madness, survival and growth. London: Whurr.

Freedman AM, Kaplan HI and Saddock BJ (1975) Comprehensive Textbook of Psychiatry. Baltimore, MD: Williams and Wilkins.

Gardener WH (ed.) (1953) Gerard Manley Hopkins, Poems and Prose. London: Penguin.

Groome TH (2002) What Makes Us Catholic, Eight Gifts for Life. San Francisco: HarperCollins.

Johnston W (1995) Mystical Theology: the science of love. London: HarperCollins.

McAlear R (1999) Healing. Rochester, NY: Association of Christian Therapists.

O'Brien E (1964) The Essential Plotinus. New York: The American Library of World Literature Inc., Mentor Books.

O'Shea R (1971) On Trial for Hope. Melbourne: Advocate Press.

Thompson F (1960) Poems of Francis Thompson. London: Oxford University Press.

Sophrony A (2002) The Tablet. March 11.

Surgeon General (1999) Report of the Surgeon General, Executive Summary. Department of Health and Human Services, US Public Health Service.

Wilber K (1985) No Boundary: Eastern and Western approaches to personal growth. Boston and London: Shambhala.

CHAPTER 11

Epiphanies

PETER WILKIN

Peter Wilkin is:

> a psychiatric nurse, crafting my practice in primary care – I belong to no particular therapeutic school, nor do I employ any specific technique – I place my trust in the other person to let me know where and how I need to be. I am driven by beauty: raging seas and scowling mountains; haunting melodies and heart-stopping works of art; of poetry that echoes deeply around my soul – and the beauty of people ... some of whom I have known; others whom I will never know.

Spiritual revelations from the body of psychiatry

> Remember your epiphanies written on green oval leaves, deeply deep, copies to be sent if you died to all the great libraries of the world.
>
> From *Ulysses* (Joyce, 1968: 141–144)

Introduction

The 'It' of psychiatry is unequivocally medical. It is a powerful, masculine-based economy that employs, seduces, profiteers, fixes and controls. Conversely, spirituality is often dismissed by psychiatric providers as merely moonshine: too groundless to have any real significance. Yet the spiritual drifts through us all, surfacing each time we are emotionally stirred. Sometimes, as we engage deeply with others, we become acutely aware of these spiritual stirrings. And, when such a coming together of

150

emotions reaches a climax, there is an evanescent moment of glory and discovery. In the words of James Joyce's protagonist, 'the object achieves its epiphany' (Joyce, 1963: 213).

The psychiatric climate – awash with strong feelings and emotionally charged relationships – provides the best growing conditions for the epiphanic moment to flourish and burst forth. Finding time to reflect and make some sense of our epiphanies leads us to our own inner wisdom and a more colourful picture of what is. After having developed this concept in detail, recorded illustrations of my own psychiatric epiphanies lead you to the end point of this text. From there, it is up to you ...

There came a day at summer's full

Glorious, most worshipful and heavenly summertime! Life was wide open and the unexplainable difference of Sunday chimed within me. Predictably early, I ambled towards my late shift and a lyrical feeling hummed gently through my veins. The afternoon sun burned into my cheeks and I closed my eyes for a few moments as I walked. Glowing red from the inside, my eyelids drank in the heat and a smile broke from the depths of my schooldays. I dared walk no further without opening my eyes – and rightly so. Just three or four more footsteps would surely have seen me striding into the lane-side nettles.

The path leading up to the road was powder grey and strangely quiet. No one else was coming or going. I reached the driveway and suddenly became aware of the oppressive heat; the nonsense of my clothes; the persecutory knot of my tie. A narrow green lawn like a moat around a castle stood between me and the crumbling red bricks of the glowering asylum. A breeze whispered by, momentarily cooling my face and, in its aftermath, a scented waft from the hybrid tea roses in the flowerbeds. A few flecks of dust powdered my mouth and I blew them away, wetting my lips and tasting the salty crystals of sweat upon them.

As I crossed the gardens I saw a lone figure sitting on a bench, laughing with no one. I knew that she was Maya and that she was 26 years of age. Her flimsy cotton frock broadcast her innocence. A pastel green ribbon hung loosely from her raddled hair and she clutched a badly clothed dolly in the crook of her arm, her head tilted and gently resting on the doll's head. She spoke softly and then listened to a voice that I could not hear. I was next to her now, yet she seemed unaware of my presence. 'Oh! No! No! No!' She started to rock slowly back and forth and began to sob, 'Oh! No! I can't leave my baby.' I stood by the ward door and dallied in the charade of searching for my key. Her frock was ice blue; her skin was so real and pale. She smelled sweetly of talcum powder and I wanted desperately to hold her and kiss the tears from her eyes. Yet my heart raced with fear at the very thought of approaching her. Heavy with the ghost of her hope, I pressed my key into the lock and closed the door between us – forever.

As my senses came home, realization followed on. Maya's helpless distress had touched me deeply and I had been paralysed by both the desire and fear of discovery. Despite my longing to comfort her tenderly, I could not. I stood naked and ashamed – useless and stripped of all my knowing how to be, before finally hiding my bareness behind the locked door of the ward. In this one ineffable, humbling moment the kudos that I had carried as a psychiatric nurse as a mingler among schizophrenics (sic) and the downright dangerous (sic) – had collapsed in a heap. Confronted by my internal deity, the haughty swagger that had publicized my designs as bravehearted mender of mad people had been reduced to a shameful skulk. Nursing, it seems, can be painful – and, at that moment in time, I was hurting real bad. It is perhaps significant that I remember very little else of that day other than my private disgrace at not only feeling unable to be with Maya but, also, my hasty retreat in order to escape my own anxiety.

Within the indolence that hangs in psychiatry's corridors and communities lie spores of becoming ... embryos in the womb of time waiting to germinate and unfold into moments of revelation. Like the phantoms and dim dreams that haunt Keats' Ode,[1] they hover, waiting to be summoned from the unconscious of every psychiatric giver and taker. Yet many such spiritual manifestations fail to break through into the light of consciousness. They are terminated by a host who is unprepared for such a sublime experience, or they wither and die – stillborn as the egg breaks.

The rhetoric of my opening story captures just one of those transient, allegorical moments that have punctuated my whole psychiatric career. Artless and unrehearsed – like a storm brewing – an unremarkable stroll through the hospital grounds climaxed like lightning in my innards. Bereft of sensical thought I felt only the sensation that the heavens had drawn breath within me. For the first time in my brief experience (I was a first-year student nurse), psychiatry had become more than just a scripted role in a godless drama. The dim religious light that shone darkly through the high ward windows had become a heavenly slanted light that beamed down and illuminated a huge cathedral of caring.[2]

---

[1] 'Ode on Indolence', John Keats: the complete poems, 3rd edn. London: Penguin Classics, 1988.

[2] Credit for the metaphors in this sentence must be attributed, first, to Emily Dickinson (1961) for her poem, 'There's a certain slant of light'. The imagery conjured by 'cathedrals of caring' was inspired by Phil Barker during a recent interview that we collaborated on: Barker P and Wilkin P (2002) A conversation with Phil Barker. Sacred Space 3(4): 15–23.

Casting off the shackles of psychiatry

As psychiatry has evolved, it has been invested with more and more meaning. Everyone who has been touched by the phenomenon – no matter how lightly, no matter how passively – has contributed a building block to the empire that it has become. It is a huge, human warehouse, home to two tribes: the psychiatrizers and the psychiatrized. Manufactured to explain and contain the whole gamut of human suffering, psychiatry has become hyper-real: realer than the actual individual experience (Baudrillard, 1983: 2). The tabloid headlines, the graphically beautiful skuldruggery of the pharmaceutical advertisements and the ever-expanding *Diagnostic and Statistical Manual of Mental Disorders* – all powerful ingredients which, when pitched together in the same pot, synergize into a propaganda that society dutifully seems to swallow. Such sophisticated jiggery-pokery has painted a vivid picture of psychiatry that has come to life; the representation has finally replaced the actual. Regrettably, this web of deceit stretches the length and breadth of the field, trapping both professionals and public alike. The metropolis of psychiatry creeps insidiously outwards, constructing diagnostic suburbs on the brownfields of people's lived experiences. Society is being pre-programmed to react in a particular way to an ever-widening number of life difficulties. With a script that is so hard to resist, spontaneity and creativity gradually give way to a discourse that covers just about every eventuality.

As a psychiatric nurse, I stand with a foot in both camps. By the very nature of my position, I have been psychiatrized. I am governed by the legislation that directs me and cloistered by the medical culture that surrounds me. I have also become a psychiatrizer! Each time I engage with an emotionally distressed other I reinforce all that has doubtless gone before: the doctor's diagnosis, the chemical reaction and the sick role that one has to accept in order to be processed along the psychiatric conveyor belt. That is a fact that does not sit comfortably, and I have to try and make some sense of that without sliding into cosy rationalization.

For me, psychiatry started out as a journey into the unknown. In the early days of my nurse training it offered me an apprenticeship geared towards the development of technical competence. I learned about symptoms and treatments and how to categorize and, at times, control the other. Gradually, the metaphors I had thrown overboard floated back on the tide and I began to haul them out of the water. Instead of turning up for work at the beginning of a shift to put on my white coat and encourage sanity, I began to celebrate madness and difference. I discovered what Homi Bhabha has called the 'liminal space' (although I did not know it as such then): a space where I could consciously deflex my organizational muscles and, quite simply, 'be' with an 'other' (Bhabha, 1994: 3–4).

Adopting an agendaless pose, I discovered, released me enough from the disabling and objectifying practices that beleaguer all healthcare employees (Wilkin, 2001: 119). Even among the striated spaces of 21st-century psychiatry it is possible to find a smooth space where the interval between entering and leaving offers a de-territorialized space of potential liberation (Fox, 1999: 202–204). Only in such spaces – created when scientific principles are surrendered and meta-narratives resisted – can the spiritual emerge from the actual.

Spirituality and human becoming

Emotional distress is a soulful experience, yet the spiritual vapours that permeate all of life's struggles are frequently reduced and converted to a symptom of the psychiatric problem. Each time human suffering is medically and cognitively eradicated, the developmental process of human becoming is simultaneously arrested. The essence of all human feeling is spiritually flavoured. Spirituality is the agony and the jouisance that form the poles of our circular existence. It is the stuff of our suffering and the distillation of all our hope.

In my capacity as a psychiatric nurse, it is my own spiritual emergence – fed by my contact with all that is other – that fills me with the emptiness to accommodate the spirit of that other. Human becoming is a gradual process that is punctuated only occasionally by a sudden spurt of growth. These bolting moments 'unbandage the soul' and expose the unthought known within us all. As Emily Dickinson declares:

> The soul has moments of Escape –
> When bursting all the doors –
> She dances like a Bomb, abroad,
> And swings upon the Hours.

> (From 'The soul has bandaged moments', Dickinson, 1961)

And it is Emily Dickinson whose poetry forges meaning deeper than any scientific equation, who leads us 'full music on' into the moment of revelation itself, as the spiritual collision:

> Deals – One – Imperial – Thunderbolt –
> That scalps your naked Soul –
> When Winds take Forests in their Paws –
> The Universe – is still –

> (From 'He fumbles at your soul', Dickinson, 1961)

From the lightning flash that suddenly strikes your soul emerges a sense of breathless waiting – a brooding period of incubation – before the light finally shines from within.

In a tradition that is home to so many diverse cultures and conflicting agendas, there is a currency that is familiar to us all – a spiritual economy that pervades the whole psychiatric marketplace. Irrespective of our designated 'mental' roles, we are all just as likely to witness, 'The fairies dance and Christ ... nailed to the cross' (Whitehead, 1978: 337). Spirituality is our only means of becoming. And such becoming reaches its peak at the moment of epiphany. Through these spiritual windows 'we can see the limitations of our current scientific knowledge and in some cases restore to ourselves some sense of humility and of wonder' (Morrison, 2000).

Epiphanies: the most delicate and evanescent moments

In the words of Stephen Daedalus, an epiphany is 'a sudden spiritual manifestation, whether in the vulgarity of speech or of gesture or in a memorable phrase of the mind itself' (Joyce, 1963: 211). Yet from within the genre of James Joyce's writings, this concept of the epiphany seems to occupy the middle ground. In *Dubliners*, Joyce's first major published work, he offers us a sequence of short stories – full of trivial significance which, collectively, become a metaphor for the spiritual and moral paralysis of a city. One such example is taken from the concluding story, 'The Dead'. In it, Joyce describes the indescribable sublimity of Gabriel Conway's spiritual meltdown, as his senses penetrate deeply through the crust of a rapidly fragmenting world to a land of both quick and dead:

> His soul swooned slowly as he heard the snow falling faintly through the universe and faintly falling, like the descent of their last end, upon all the living and the dead.
>
> Joyce (1992a: 225)

This thought-enchanted silence transports Gabriel – sum and substance – to a numinous place of knowing. Structure has capsized and, with it, the differentiation between the 'I' and the 'it'. The epiphanic moment is nomadic and strictly I-Thou, as 'only when every means has collapsed does the meeting come about' (Buber, 1958: 25).

In his later works, Joyce's abstraction of the epiphany undergoes a metamorphosis. Much like Benson's (Benson, 1993: 1–10) concept of being 'aesthetically absorbed', Joyce's protagonist in the *Stephen Hero* text employed Aquinas' aesthetic theory to describe 'the revelatory climax of aesthetic apprehension' (Mahaffey, 1990: 190). Here, the birthing of the epiphany relies on the spiritual eye adjusting its focus to discover the supreme quality of beauty – the 'whatness' – in an object. Only in such a spiritually aroused state can we genuinely discover the radiance that shines within 'the soul of the commonest object' (Joyce, 1963: 213).

Published posthumously in 1944, the *Stephen Hero* manuscript became the chrysalis and imago for Joyce's (1992b) *A Portrait of the Artist as a Young Man*. Again, the epiphany underwent further transformation and, according to Mahaffey, represented 'a rare balance of spirit and matter ... an evenness of apprehension illustrated by the commingling of light and darkness in Shelley's image of a "fading coal"' (Mahaffey, 1990: 192). While Mahaffey's explanation seems plausible enough, it seems to deny the thunder of the epiphanic implosion. Such awe-inspiring moments penetrate our souls like a Bach toccata booms into the roof. Yet, as quickly as the echo fades, these moments 'pass away'. But this is a death with a difference that wakes the 'heart in hiding' and stirs a 'fire that breaks' within.[3] The dying of the epiphanic moment – like all deaths do – leaves us with an aftershock, a revelation, a discovery of just one of the host of shapeless spirits that dance and tap lightly on our souls. It is a sublime encounter with the 'other' where 'the space between breaths becomes one soul' (Clarkson, 1997: 2).

Epiphanies: a communion with otherness

We cannot have a spiritual experience in isolation. We need the 'object' of a human being, a mountain, a tiger, a symphony or a god to light the blue touch-paper of those dormant spirits within us. Bollas describes such a process, quite simply, as 'spiritual communication', where we become 'receptive to the intelligent breeze of the other who moves through us, to affect us, shaping within us the ghost of that spirit when it is long gone' (Bollas, 1992: 63). For Bollas, 'being a character' involves receptivity to a spirit-swapping that 'conjugate(s) into meaning-laden experience' (Bollas, 1992: 65).

Taking Jung's concept of synchronicity as his exploratory engine, Peat calls on the poet Hopkins' terms 'inscape' and 'instress'[4] to describe the

---

[3] Both these short phrases are taken from Gerard Manley Hopkins' poem 'The Windhover'. While the poem itself is epiphanic, it is the beauty of Christ that creates such breathtaking poetic moments that it celebrates. (Selected Poetry: Gerard Manley Hopkins. Oxford: Oxford University Press, 1998.)

[4] Hopkins' concept of inscape is similar to Stephen's explanation of epiphany to Cranly in *Stephen Hero*, in that it describes the 'whatness' of an object. Unlike James Joyce's epiphanies, though, Hopkins' term is fundamentally religious. By 'instress', Hopkins referred to the impulse that emanated from and transported the inscape of an object into the soul.

fusion of inner and outer experiences that manifest as seamless moments of knowing (Peat, 2002). Rather than seeking 'a direct causal involvement' between the two, he sees it more as a harmonious blending of energies and spirits until there is only 'darkness within darkness. The gateway to all understanding' (Lao-tzu, 2000: No. 1). Like a nerve impulse leaping from axon to neuron, the inscape of an object is transmitted into the soul of the beholder. When the pregnancy that saturates Glen Coe frightens the joy out of me; and the gentle weeping of Beck's guitar causes me to cry tears from the core of my being – these are the spiritual synapses triggered when I open up my self and surrender to inscape.

Unlike the Christian interpretation of epiphany, where the receiver is consumed in a beam of blinding light, Paris offers us the pagan alternative of 'everyday epiphanies', where 'you sense Aphrodite both in your orgasms and when you are gardening' (Paris, 1997: 95). Rather than confirming the existence of God, her hypothesis of epiphanies is more akin to the early Joycean construct that involves 'casual, unostentatious, even unpleasant moments' (Ellman, 1982: 83), which are 'part and parcel of everyday life' (Paris, 1997: 93). These are the moments that have suddenly engulfed me, at intervals, during my psychiatric nursing career. Though the spiritual has become my constant companion, it is these epiphanies – these spiritual shocks – that have brought about the greatest edification.

Epiphanies: elusive phantoms of delight

Whenever these epiphanies do descend, they are brimming with wisdom that spills and rushes through our bodies. Yet no mesh is fine enough to trap these 'spots of time'.[5] Such moments, like fairies at the bottom of the garden, are beyond capture. Adrift and 'uncertain as under sea', their ethereal nature renders them elusive and difficult to hypostasize. Soaked only in the spindrift of this breaking wave, how can we ever hope to journalize our epiphanies? How can we begin to make sense of them and truly understand them?

Having experienced such a radical, intersubjective state, one is left with a tantalizing summary of the full story. Epiphanies are open sesames that lead us to the unthought treasures of knowing within us all. The search for such meaning, of course, lies further upstream from the point of the encounter. Sometimes, the self-knowing to be gained from these experiences is swept by the current of time to surface an age away. On other

---

[5] 'Spots of time', taken from William Wordsworth's lengthy poem 'Prelude', refer to the recollection of significant childhood experiences that serve to spiritually nourish and regenerate us. Prelude: Book XII, Imagination and taste, how impaired and restored. The Works of William Wordsworth. Hertfordshire: Wordsworth Editions, 1994.

occasions, we stumble upon it peering out from under the very next stepping stone. The lamp that casts most lighting on these internal moments is undoubtedly a reflective one. Whether purposefully engaged with a chosen other (e.g. a supervisor, an emotionally distressed person or a trusted colleague) or by oneself, the doorway to self-understanding sits clearly within the process of reflection.

Having made sense of them, recording our epiphanies becomes a vital, yet oft-neglected, responsibility. These big moments that spring from our souls provide revenue that serves to connect us all together. While textbooks explain and models direct and contain, the spiritual gives us the 'is'. Though I will choose the medium to deliver a description of my epiphanies, you will inevitably tune in via your own senses. This chapter becomes the gap and all the stories are metaphors – waiting in anticipation for you to step into that space. All of them are doors for you to enter; to catch a glimpse of creation and the grave; to feel my flesh – the goose bumps raised in angst and celebration.

I have little else to write, other than 'make of my epiphanies what you will'. I have surrendered them to you on the following pages just as they happened. And, like Joyce, I have resisted all temptation to lead you beyond the glorious moment into detailed explication. They are yours to re-author and rewrite with your own special spiritual ink.

Epiphany 1: Anna

When Anna arrived on the ward I took an immediate liking to her. I was on duty the day she was admitted and recall her announcement the following day that she was to marry Derek, our charge nurse – despite not yet having shared this information with him. The wedding was to take place at Ely Cathedral (which was Anna's home city) and she was planning to leave the ward to organize her wedding dress, the bridesmaids' outfits and the flowers. I was to be the groom's best man!

When he learned of Anna's proposals, Derek took it all in his stride. He was 26 years of age; she would soon be 44. She was quite a slender woman, with thick, long, red hair that contrasted violently with her lime green suit – the only exterior clothing that she seemed to possess. While I apologize in advance for the judgemental comment, it is necessary to describe her as not particularly attractive. She had a pronounced squint, decorated with turquoise eye shadow and corrected only marginally by the plate-glass lenses in her tortoiseshell spectacles. Her shoes, I remember, were scuffed and a dull cherry red.

Anna never did make it to the shops that day. She was pronounced too irresponsible and too vulnerable to leave the ward and was subsequently restrained from doing so, courtesy of the Mental Health Act. Anna was livid – and we all suffered the backlash, until she was silenced by the doctor's divine potion of paraldehyde syrup.[6]

It was now 8.15pm and, a full three hours after Anna had swallowed her punishment (for that is how I interpreted it), the reek of this abusive juice hung heavily in every corner of the female dormitory. Visiting time had come and gone and, despite her plans to invite 'over 200 people' to her wedding reception, not one person had called to comfort her. The bedroom door was ajar and, with a cup of tea in my hand, I cautiously announced my arrival. There was no definite response, although I thought I heard a stirring from the direction of Anna's bed. I slowly made my way down past three or four empty beds, calling out 'Hello!' once more.

As I reached Anna's cubicle, the curtain that served as a flimsy excuse for privacy was half drawn. I spoke her name softly before taking the final few steps to her humble berth. Still fully clothed, she raised herself to a sitting position, showing no emotion at all. The vivid blue of her eye shadow was stained with dark rivulets of mascara that had carried her earlier tears. Her glasses were nowhere to be seen and the combined effects of her strabismus and the powerful drug prevented her from focusing. I noticed her lips ... the smudged vermilion glow and the parched cracks that had begun to crust over. I moved closer to place the tea on her locker and the slightest hint of her heavy perfume momentarily filtered through the odour of paraldehyde.

It was then that I really saw her ... it was then that her beauty touched me ... and in this instant, she was a child to be read nursery rhymes ... and a lover to be fed sugar-dipped strawberries. And I sat with her in the torrential rains of a summer storm – and smelled her womanness – and slew the dragons that caged her with their fiery breath. And then, in another ticking of the clock, every last droplet of shame that had ever coursed through me flamed a blush that burned my whole being.

Epiphany 2: Tom

Although I had worked in the community for nigh on 15 years, I had been approached to work a night shift on one of the acute admission wards. 'We are desperate!' I was told. I rationalized that it would be an interesting experience. 'I will do it!' I replied.

---

[6] Paraldehyde is a nervous system depressant that has a pronounced sedative effect. It has a very disagreeable odour and actually melts plastic syringes! If given by injection it can cause tissue damage and, if given orally, can irritate the throat and stomach. It is also used as a preservative in the manufacture of synthetic resins!

Friday, 10.25pm. Closed doors and curtains the colour of mulberries kept all the madness inside the hospital. One of the patients (for that is what they most certainly were) had wheeled in a tea trolley from the kitchen. On it sat a row of mugs filled with steaming hot chocolate. A second patient had brought in a white dinner plate stacked full of very ordinary biscuits. I recall I was the only nurse sat within a small group of these patients. A few of them were poking fun at each other and laughing loudly as though everything was fine. Some of the others grinned reluctantly in feigned alliance.

I was approached by the ward sister, whom I did not know. She said that Tom was preparing to go to bed and I was next on the rota to 'special' him. I had a vague idea of what would be involved. She said he had been placed on 'close observations' and it was crucial that I never strayed more than an arm's length away from him. I read his notes. He had a medical diagnosis of schizophrenia and he had attempted to jump out of a ward window only two days previously.

I introduced myself to Tom. He smiled but did not reply. He was putting on his pyjamas. I outlined my brief and confessed my virginal surveillance status. I had no need – I knew that he knew. He still did not speak. He went to the bathroom and urinated. I went with him and watched. I was riddled with anxiety and awkwardness. We returned to his bed and he climbed in. I pulled up a chair and sat by his bedside to begin my vigil.

The low beam of the dormitory night light – which I had been told 'must stay on' – enabled me to read. I opened my book – and all the words scattered and hid. I closed my book and gazed upon my charge. He was restless and struggling to settle. He turned towards me, eyes closed ... and gripped the bedclothes tightly in his hand ... blankets too rough for comfort. I saw his face and smelled his rank odour ... I was his sentinel – yet sat in his dungeon. He was the one with needles in his eyes, so desperate to jump from this mortal coil. Yet it was I – in the black hole of my yawning insignificance – who heard the death knell ringing.

Observations

In the I of the night
By the it of the bed
I gaze on an other
Who plans to be dead

Crowned on the cross
A king with no plea
Condemned by his difference
To the medic and me

Hospital pyjamas
Cerulean blue
Mental disorder
Detained on a '2'

His voices are calling
No sound can I hear
I could reach out and touch him
Yet I feel nowhere near

The rough of his stubble
The damp of his sweat
The smoke of his breathing
How close can I get?

There is me on a chair
There is he by my side
It is he who is doomed
It is I who have died

(Peter Wilkin)

Epiphany 3: Aaron

Aaron was devastated and devoid of all hope. We had sat together for the best part of an hour as he tried to make some sense of his partner's recent suicide. He had returned from work one evening to an empty house. The following morning her body was discovered in a nearby wood. I could taste Aaron's agony and contrition. I had no sense of myself, as his calvary consumed us like a death mist.

As he spoke, his words broke the spell of that I-Thou moment. I became acutely aware of me and my fear, as Aaron announced his intention to kill himself. He would find a secluded spot and take a massive overdose of tablets. I knew that Aaron meant what he was saying – and I knew that it was vital that I did nothing – nothing other than being. I wanted Aaron to be in hospital. I wanted to relinquish all responsibility and hand it over to the psychiatric doctors and nurses on the ward. But it was only my need and most certainly not what Aaron wanted. He was adamant that he wanted to die and, once again, I took hold of his intentions with the whole of my being. Our meeting drew to a close. Broken from the trance of such an emotional session I could think of nothing better to say than, 'I will be here for you at exactly the same time again next week.' Aaron acknowledged my awkward comment with non-verbally expressed futility, yet I sensed heartfelt thanks in his eyes as he rose from his chair. We clasped hands tighter than usual and he left.

I thought of Aaron often over the next three days. On the fourth day I returned to base and picked up a telephone message. It simply said, 'See you as arranged, Aaron.'

Aaron welcomed me with a smile that signified much more than a mere greeting – and proceeded to share his amazing experience with me. He had left our session and gone home to prepare for his own suicide. He had written a note and then driven, at midnight, to a small isolated carpark on the edge of town. There, he had consumed copious amounts of whisky and a cocktail of tablets. He had vague recollections of waking in the daylight and seeing 'an angel's face'. His next memory was the gradual gathering together of his thoughts as he found himself at home, fully dressed, in bed. It was all a complete mystery to him how he had arrived there. His suicide note was unopened on the kitchen table where he had left it. His car – which he went to pick up a day later – was still in the car park. It was unlocked and the radio was missing.

A clamouring silence descended upon us – consuming us – like an enchanting tale. We had entered the same story; become the characters ... knew the script backwards. Pulses synchronized, a whisper of foreverness shivered through our heartbeat. The bloodless shadow that had blacked out Aaron's soul had lifted. A soft light waxed, now – deeply down – incubating the 'tender leaves of hope'. He was different ... we never questioned 'why?'

References

Baudrillard J (1983) Simulations. New York: Semiotext(e).

Benson C (1993) The Absorbed Self: pragmatism, psychology and aesthetic experience. Hertfordshire: Harvester Wheatsheaf.

Bhabha HK (1994) The Location of Culture. London: Routledge.

Bollas C (1992) Being a Character: psychoanalysis and self experience. London: Routledge.

Buber M (1958) I and Thou. Edinburgh: T & T Clark.

Clarkson P (1997) The sublime in psychoanalysis and archetypal psychotherapy In Clarkson P (ed.) On the Sublime in Psychoanalysis, Archetypal Psychology and Psychotherapy. London: Whurr.

Dickinson E (1961) The Complete Poems of Emily Dickinson. Boston, MA: Back Bay Books.

Ellman R (1982) James Joyce. Oxford: Oxford University Press.

Fox NJ (1999) Beyond Health: postmodernism and embodiment. London: Free Association Books.

Joyce J (1963) Stephen Hero. New York: New Directions.

Joyce J (1968) Ulysses. London: Penguin Classics.

Joyce J (1992a) Dubliners. London: Penguin Classics.

Joyce J (1992b) A Portrait of the Artist as a Young Man. London: Minerva.

Lao-tzu (2000) Tao Te Ching: the book of the way (translated by Stephen Mitchel). London: Kyle Cathie.

Mahaffey V (1990) Joyce's shorter works. In Attridge D (ed.) The Cambridge Companion to James Joyce. Cambridge: Cambridge University Press.

Morrison A (2000) Celtic spirituality and the gift of second sight. Available at: http://www.tartans.com/articles/secondsight3.html (accessed 5 August 2002).

Paris G (1997) Everyday epiphanies. In Clarkson P (ed.) On the Sublime in Psychoanalysis, Archetypal Psychology and Psychotherapy. London: Whurr.

Peat FD (2002) Synchronicity: the speculum of inscape and landscape. Available at: http://www.fdavidpeat.com/bibliography/essays/synch.htm (accessed 16 August 2002).

Whitehead AN (1978) Process and Reality. New York: The Free Press.

Wilkin P (2001) From medicalisation to hybridization: a postcolonial discourse for psychiatric nurses. Journal of Psychiatric and Mental Health Nursing 8(2): 115–120.

PART FOUR
Healings

It is more necessary for the soul to be healed than the body; for it is better to die than to live ill.

Epictetus

Believe to the end, even if all men went astray and you were left the only one faithful; bring your offering even then and praise God in your loneliness.

Dostoevsky

The inner voice – the human compulsion when deeply distressed to seek healing counsel within ourselves, and the capacity within ourselves both to create this counsel and to receive it.

Alice Walker

CHAPTER 12
Heavenbound

NIKKI SLADE

Nikki Slade is an actress and musician and has appeared in repertory theatre, at the Royal National Theatre and in the West End. However:

> I truly believe that destiny had other plans for me, as my chapter fully explains. Upon leaving the hospital, my life path shifted to an exploration of voice and sound. Although I thoroughly enjoyed appearing at the Young Vic in a northern soul musical, singing solo at Pizza on the Park jazz room and singing in my own band in Covent Garden, eventually the voicework became the most meaningful aspect of my life. To this day, my company 'Free the Inner Voice' flourishes well in a broad spectrum of fields including children, general public, mental health, business and public performance.

Nikki lives in Twickenham, England, with her partner, Yasia, who is her constant friend, companion and ally on the spiritual path.

> Unmistakeable on the front of the train, instead of 'Upminster' was the word, 'Heavenbound'. My spiritual journey had already started, and it is not over yet.

The original experience

In February 1989 I was living in Wandsworth, London, earning my keep in a delicatessen up the road from my home. I was in a stagnant relationship, and it reflected my feelings at the time that all was empty and meaningless. 'There must be more to life than this,' was the recurring phrase within me – but what?

Although I was qualified as an actress and singer, my professional life was going through a dry patch. I had had fulfilling periods in this field, but somehow I knew that this was not the solution to my despondency. As I went to work each day, each sandwich I had to make for each customer seemed more and more futile. When I returned home in the evenings, the effects of alcohol were no longer as comforting as before. However, I had recently been introduced to chanting and meditation in a very strong yogic tradition. One day, feeling particularly low, I began chanting some of the sacred mantras I had been introduced to at the meditation centre that month. I decided to make it a regular practice.

I would go home each lunch break and turn on the chanting tape and sing along with it. I didn't notice any particular difference in my state at first, but three days into the practice, something happened. I began to feel much lighter, less bothered by the menial work I thought I was doing – in fact it became quite fun. After chanting I felt warmth in my heart and a friendliness that I automatically wanted to share with the customers. I began to take quite an interest in what they wanted in their sandwiches, offering them all sorts of combinations. I would begin to ask about how they were and what they were planning to do that day. One day I felt so merry that I began to feel very connected to the radio playing in the shop. I would tap into the news and hear it as if some of the points were specially meant for my ears. A report about the ozone layer seemed particularly meaningful. When an unassuming builder came in for his sandwich, I began to ask him what he felt about the ozone layer, as if we were all personally responsible for it. He looked at me quizzically, not sure whether I was genuine or a potential fruitcake! I no longer cared what anybody thought, because I was becoming happier and happier inside.

After one week, things around me began to shift radically, or at least my perception of them did. As I chanted, my little cat, Bluesy, began to communicate with me in an unusual way. She would sit by the telephone as I was singing, and I would say to her in a 'cat voice', '*di di doo tinkatink doo*'. She would stare hard back at me and all of a sudden the telephone would jangle. It seemed that she was playing with me. 'Did you make that telephone jangle?' I'd say to her. She'd blink her eyes back at me and the same thing would happen again. My heart started to pump harder and faster. This was a phenomenon I couldn't explain.

I then went into my bedroom where I saw in the litterbin two demo tapes, very special song projects that I was working on, which I knew I would never have thrown away. How could this be? I was spooked!

I returned to work and then it really started. I looked at the cheese counter and all the parsley and spinach began to dance – just like the little people in *Tom Thumb*. I found it very entrancing and amusing. The shop assistant, Michelle, turned to me and all of a sudden I could see her resemblance to a creature from the ape kingdom. It was like my eyes were playing tricks as she ate a banana in front of me. I managed to suppress my laughter at this baboon-like figure when the proprietor asked me to arrange the potatoes in baskets at the front of the shop. I had a sudden impulse to make them look beautiful, because that's how I felt and I wanted to express it. I began to fold pink tissue paper into little flowers and placed them between each potato, much to the dismay of Anthony, who said, 'What on earth do you think you are doing? You can only put that paper among the apples.' I didn't care. I was in bliss.

Later, I left the shop and walked down the hill to see the most incredible sunset. It was so exquisite that I felt it was an extension of my body and all was ecstasy. I couldn't believe that I was experiencing something so extraordinary without the use of drugs or alcohol. I really believed I'd cracked the secret of life. I went home to my partner, Liz, who couldn't believe how joyful I was; she was definitely uplifted and infected by my energy. It was the weekend, and one I will never forget.

That Saturday, I was due to go and try on clothes that I was going to wear to present a fashion show in Cardiff on the Monday. My friend Davina, who had given me the job, invited me to her home in Battersea. I decided to take a walk in Battersea Park en route, and it was there that I had the most euphoric experience.

In the park, the duality of my perception dissolved and I felt absolutely connected to every tree, bird, dog, lake, person, in fact to Nature in her entirety, all in one moment. I waved at everybody without any fear and, to my amazement, everyone waved back. This felt better than an orgasm! I was experiencing musical symphonies arising inside me that were beyond a human orchestra. 'Wow! What's happening to me?' I said to myself.

Eventually I arrived at the house and went to ring the bell, number 25. There was no reply. 'Hmm, that's odd,' I thought. I kept ringing, but eventually gave up and went home, from where I rang Davina. 'Where were you?' I asked. 'I'm here,' she said. 'At number 25.'

I knew this was odd, and was definitely down to my present state of mind, just like the tinkling telephone (which, incidentally, had played up again as I dialled her number). That was when I heard demoniacal voices breathing and growling heavily. I was momentarily scared, but then returned to Davina's house. Her boyfriend, Leon, was there, and when he began to talk to me about cats, I had the experience that I was talking with him in another dimension, as if he had stepped out of time and I was meant to be receiving a message about my connection with the cat kingdom. Well this of course made sense, after my experience with Bluesy! That whole hour was deeply surreal.

I collected my outfit. Later, Liz and I went out to dinner with friends. As we arrived at Verity's, I looked at Liz and saw her face beginning to change. A lightning mark suddenly appeared in the middle of her forehead, and her face began to crumble in front of me. I closed my eyes and shook my head, very alarmed by this illusion.

We went inside Verity's flat. As I sat around the table with my five friends, the dimensions shifted again. We were all in Egypt. Verity was dressed like a belly dancer, Caroline like a water bearer, Paul like a soldier and Chaz seemed like some kind of demon as I watched the cigarette smoke passing in and out of her mouth. I stood up at the table and banter immediately came out of my mouth, as if I was a comedian like Max Wall or Tony Hancock. Whatever I spouted had everybody in absolute hysterics, but I can't say that it was anything to do with me. It was as if something was using me as its puppet. After supper, I began to feel immensely 'flower-powery' and wanted to hug everybody, but Liz sensed that there was something 'off' with me, and soon afterwards insisted on taking me home.

That night I had another extraordinary experience. I began to hear tapping on the window beside our bed. I heard the voice of my first partner at college. Her name was Holly and I thought she wanted to come in. I saw with a sudden intuition who she was. Once again the dimension reverted to Egypt and a time when we had been lovers, only then I was male, not female. Holly was tied to a stake and was being repeatedly beaten by soldiers. I saw my father as their leader, the one who had authorized this barbarism. The dimension dissolved and my inner voice revealed that this was why my father and Holly never got on well together. My father, as a rule, liked all my friends, but in this case he couldn't accept her. I was then shown why Holly used to harm herself by scratching her arms with sharp blades. It was all connected to the scenes in Egypt and unresolved karma from that time.

By now the night had passed, and it was the early hours of Monday morning. Liz slept obliviously beside me as I began to feel an incredible heat and juddering at the base of my spine. I was really scared. I thought I was going to explode.

I jumped out of bed, and could only walk doubled over. I made my way to the kitchen, as I needed air. Opening the back door, I was met by the elements. There was the most incredible storm, one of biblical proportions. Lightning cracked and flashed above my head, and the sound of thunder went crashing through my ears. I forced the door shut against the wind as the cat began to circle my legs. All I could hear then was a mad hissing sound, as if Bluesy was a snake lassoing her way around me. I looked in the mirror and my hair was standing on end as if an electric current ran through it. My eyes looked like those of someone who had seen a ghost. 'Matt will look after you,' a voice said. 'He will be your guardian angel for the day. Do not let him leave your side.'

Spookily, at that moment, Matt, the make-up artist for the fashion day, arrived to escort me, as we had previously arranged. Matt was a beautiful, effeminate man, who at that time had long curly locks, dyed bright purple. He did indeed resemble an angel that day. I was told inside that I was about to embark on an incredible journey. I went to Liz's bedside and whispered in her ear, 'I'm going now, and I might be some time.' 'Don't be silly, I'll see you later,' she said, 'it's only Wales.' But I knew something different.

Matt and I walked through the streets of Wandsworth, and in that moment Wandsworth was ecstasy. I felt as if my feet were six inches off the ground, and I was levitating like some Indian saddhu. I felt like we were in some religious painting depicting a chariot ridden by windswept angels. As we walked into East Putney station, the train pulled in and to my amazement instead of 'Upminster' on the front, it said 'Heavenbound'. Looking round the carriage, I thought, 'These people must all be on their way to Heaven, just like me!' It was a wonderful feeling.

It was not long before we arrived at High Street Kensington, but my awareness was timeless. I looked at my watch and giggled at its face and its impossible attempt to measure the passing of minutes. It seemed only a moment before we were then stepping into the hotel where we, along with 50 fashion models and crew, were meeting the coach to Cardiff. I picked up a newspaper, and couldn't believe how out of date the headlines were. I suddenly realized, intuitively again, that I'd gone back from the future, just like HG Wells' *The Time Machine*. As we got onto the coach, I laughed at the shows playing at West End theatres. They all sounded incredibly out of date. I was having the experience of being from a time much further ahead in the future, and I could slip in and out of normal dimensional reality.

Then, as we set off, the guidance started. I was asked to direct my eyes towards the pagoda of the Buddha as we drove past Battersea Park. 'Look, look,' the voice said, 'the East is joining the West. It's just starting, you'll see.' The voice added a warning, 'They tried to do it in the 1960s but there was too much drug interference.' Just then I was handed the fashion event programme. The man who gave it to me, Joe, was to become very significant over the following hours. He was the director of the event, and had a shaven head. To me, Joe had the quality of the Buddha: kind, gentle and sincere. I glanced at the programme and saw that the theme of the show was Eastern in nature (more evidence for the East–West merger). I looked up to a telly screen at the front of the coach and there was an apparition, a cross between my female meditation master (from the yogic path I had started that year) and Holly, my ex-partner. They seemed to be merged into one. Holly's surname was Lingham, and I was told from within that this was similar to 'Shiva Lingam', the masculine aspect of universal energy from the Hindu tradition. This seemed more than just a coincidence.

I was shown that through my loving earthly connection with Holly, in terms of spiritual development, I was going to move through the chakra levels, eventually to the highest, the crown chakra. This symbolic link between Holly and me was deliberately meant to reflect the supreme and also loving relationship between myself and the divine feminine, as embodied by and in my meditation master. In that moment, I realized the intention behind the resemblance between these two women, Holly and my teacher, both so precious to me.

As the coach stopped at a service station, my mind-state was continuing to expand. The sky was exquisite, and I began to wax lyrical to the entire busload of people that we all had universal bliss within us and that we were on a magical journey. As we pulled into Cardiff, the first thing I saw was a poster of the Beatles' Magical Mystery Tour, and I had an ecstatic moment, tapping into the transcendental space from which some of their songs had emerged.

After we arrived at the Conference Centre, where the fashion show was to be held, I was sent on a sandwich round with one of the helpers. As we got to the bakery, the dimensions of my mind split again and I found myself standing on a royal red carpet, surrounded by golden chariots like in the movie *Ben Hur*. I seemed to be dressed in a gold-plated uniform, and made my way to a throne at the end of the carpet as I took my bow to the Queen of that time ... But suddenly the image was shattered. 'Cheese and onion or tuna?' asked the girl beside me. 'What?' I said, as I jumped, startled to find that I was not in Rome but standing in the middle of Cardiff High Street. 'You lost it for a minute there,' she said, but I think she'd only put my behaviour down to absent-mindedness. 'I need to go for a walk,' I said. 'I'll see you in a minute.' I was determined to reconnect with the golden chariots. There were no Roman signs in the high street, however, so I decided to head for the nearest church!

Arriving at a church, I was determined to find a sign showing me how to continue this exquisite experience, but I only met with tedious reality. There were some pictures of Christian saints on the walls, but no golden chariots or red carpets. In my shirtsleeves, I began returning despondently to the Conference Centre through the pouring rain. As I got halfway there, it started again – the voice within me, guiding me into the future, to the time when my mother had already passed away. In this moment I experienced huge emotional attachments. It was so convincing, that I really believed her dead. I rang home to speak to my friend Mo and asked him if my mother was still alive. 'Of course she is,' he said. 'If you like I can phone her.' 'Please,' I said. 'It's an emergency.'

I arrived back at the Centre, altered and confused as the channelling kept coming in and out of my psyche. Abruptly, before I knew it and could take stock, I was in the auditorium, surrounded by BBC cameras, preparing for the compèring I was about to do for this well-known fashion show.

Joe, the man I had termed 'Buddha', was my technical director. He gave me a sheet listing the fashion headings. The first was called, 'Chasing the Dragon'. I froze. This was a well-known term from the 1960s for drug use. The guidance had already cautioned me and told me that this was the crucial element, blocking the life force in the time of flower power.

I had to think quickly. 'Can't we call it chasing the flower?' I said this with obvious sincerity, to the point where he couldn't object. 'Alright, if that's what you would prefer,' he replied. At which point my heart opened and I felt a song coming on. It was 'As Long As He Needs Me' from the musical, 'Oliver'.

I began to parade around, singing my heart out without realizing that I was being filmed by the BBC. Their people obviously thought I was the dress rehearsal entertainment. Then I was interrupted by a voice. 'Nikki, we really don't have time for this now. We must prepare for the show.' It was Davina.

Matt, my guardian angel, was summoned to sit with me in a small room. As the guidance had revealed that he wasn't to leave me, I would not even let the poor man go to the toilet. I looked in the mirror and began to see my mother's face in mine. I cried hysterically at the prospect of death and separation from her. I couldn't accept death as a reality that all of us face. I don't think I have ever screamed such tears of desperation, but then I was interrupted by a voice. It appeared to be coming from Matt; however, his face had suddenly been transformed into that of a Tibetan god. My eyes were drawn towards his ear, which in this vision had the most exquisite jewellery attached to its lobe. 'Listen,' the ear said, 'I am with you. Do not leave my side.'

Davina came into the room with a glass of water for me. 'No,' I replied, rejecting it, convinced that all Perrier water had a zillionth of heroin in it – its marketing attraction. 'Your parents are coming,' she said. 'It's going to take them a few hours.' 'My mother is dead,' I said. I pushed past her through the door and onto the auditorium stage, charging like Boadicea (Boudicca) in Trafalgar Square. This voice came out of me from nowhere. I saw the bewildered faces of 25 models in Eastern robes. 'This is a message for anyone who has a mother,' I called out. 'Mother Earth is weeping, and we must act now.' The people in the auditorium, camera crew included, were stunned. This was not my normal voice.

I was pulled off the stage, and had a flashback to a lifetime as a religious rights activist about to be silenced. I returned to the little room, whereupon a call came through from my mother. 'We'll be with you shortly, darling.' 'No you won't, you're dead,' I said. 'It's alright. Daddy and I will be there soon,' she said. Some hours later, my parents stood before me, my mother shaking as she smoked a cigarette. I could see the smoke moving through her skeletal form. I could see through her skin, as if looking at an X-ray. 'Stop smoking!' I screeched, 'It is going to kill you!'

The journey home was horrendous for my parents and extremely surreal for all of us. I began to be spoken to by what I still believe today to be extraterrestrial beings. They showed me a UFO ship that was watching me from above, driving along the motorway with my parents, and we were the size of a Tonka toy car, relative to them. 'Have you had enough yet Nik?' the voices said, 'You can always come home.' It occurred to me for a split second that I had been more than, and would again be more than, only Nikki Slade. She is or was a temporary experience, I began to realize. These beings were my buddies. They made me laugh in the car.

We arrived at a service station. My mother needed the toilet. I was petrified to let her out of the car in case she never came back. I watched her leave and screamed again, my father trying to control me. The force within me was so strong that I was afraid. I kept repeating, 'Through Jesus Christ our Lord. Through Jesus Christ our Lord ...' Eventually, we arrived at the family home in East Sheen. I had occasional periods of lucidity and normality, but then it would all start again. The 'ETs' were talking to me, this time in a code language. Finding a way to communicate with them, I began to tap my head in a kind of coded pattern, so as to have a conversation with them. They made me laugh so hard. 'What *is* the matter?' said my mother. 'Oh, I'm just speaking to Martians,' I replied.

My parents tried to remain calm, sipping their evening drinks. My partner, Liz, arrived, both shocked and relieved at the same time to see me in this bizarre state. Caroline from next door was also called round. I began hallucinating again, this time to the point where I felt the energy of another neighbour, Mrs Hall (although she was already deceased), entering my being! She had been an angry woman, and I felt her spirit ordering me to pick up a kitchen knife, at which point Liz – a professional nurse – knew that enough was enough. I began jumping on the bed in my red spotted nightgown. The more my father shouted at me, the more hyper I became. Our family GP was called, for the second time. Earlier I had managed to reassure her that I was perfectly alright and that I was simply chatting to Martians. However, on the second visit, she knew an ambulance was the only option.

The experience of the hospital

The ambulancemen arrived and I was convinced that their intention was to rape me, as I tapped into the terror I had felt when threatened by men in previous incarnations. I hissed violently at them and pointed my finger very accusingly at their penises. They almost refused to take me, but eventually I stopped resisting and fell into their arms. As I did so, I saw myself once again in Rome, wearing sandals. I didn't know where I was going, but the guidance revealed that I was to be locked up, because I had too much top-secret information that could be dangerous to the government. The ambulance stopped inside the gates at Long Grove Hospital in Epsom. The darkness was pitch black. I was petrified. Surely this was to be the raping ground.

Suddenly, however, I found myself in one of the medical offices. My father had been led to a neighbouring room, from where I could hear a dialogue about whether or not I should have ECT. I shot back into the Roman life and saw him as a Caesar on a muddy moor. 'You will die for this.' I wasn't sure which life I was in at that moment when the guidance said, 'Your father has saved you from the ECT. He is a good man.'

The doctors then came towards me as I shook, remembering the life when I was burnt by flames. 'Drink this,' they said. I chucked the liquid medicine at them in reply. Before I knew it, I was being carted away in a wheelchair by two nurses, who seemed to me to be like a pair of malevolent dwarves. I was taken to Ross ward, a place for the real nutters of this world. It was full of ancient men and women with barely any years of life left. It struck me as if they had been asleep for decades. I stood over the bed of an old woman with pimples. A voice spoke through me to her. 'It's alright sweetheart,' and I kissed her on the lips. Her eyes shone back out of her sunken face. 'Will you come here?' said the nurses, but I jumped like a monkey onto the curtain rail, and swung out of their reach from one rail to the next. This went on for a few minutes, but finally I surrendered. They caught me and twisted my arm and I had to give in. I saw myself in Rome, crippled and bent double, being chased by soldiers and dogs. At that moment the syringe went into my rear.

Oblivious to any visitors that I might have had, I awoke 48 hours later in a padded cell wearing a blue nightgown that wasn't mine, giddy and covered in my own excrement. I remember the tears pouring out of my eyes, but I felt no connection to them. A voice spoke to me so gently that it made me cry. 'All there is, is love, Nikki. When you see this, you will understand that none of this is real.' An unbelievable compassion arose within me. I saw everyone I'd ever known and all I felt was love. All battles were over.

That night I was moved to a different ward and the shadow voices started. Always at night they came. They were very disturbing and graphic. One stopped me from getting into the bath. It was in the plughole, and definitely capable of sucking me under. The other told me to retrieve a dead embryo from the lavatory. It was hard to sleep with such mania in my mind. 'Big Judy', my Jamaican friend, slept in the cubicle beside me.

'Are you alright?' she said as she sat over my bed. 'Go away,' I said. 'Don't rape me.' (A mix-up of dimension once again!) A burning in my body began from head to toe. 'Doctor, doctor, help me!' I said – but they could find nothing physically wrong. This was no ordinary heat. I have come to understand that this was spiritual energy doing its work, cleansing the impressions of lifetimes. I saw myself stepping out of the hospital building. It felt completely real. I was in my spotted gown once again, and three army tanks came towards me. I stood in a crucifix position as the tanks blew me apart!

The next morning I was convinced that I had awoken in Heaven. My bedclothes were crisp and I had never, as I looked in the mirror, seen my eyes so crystal blue. 'You've had an operation,' said the voice inside, 'but not the usual kind.'

I went to the dining room. I felt I could conquer the world. Suddenly my inner eye opened and there was the most beautiful sight I had ever seen. There was a radiant being in electric blue robes, with jet black hair and charcoal eyes, dripping with dew. It communed with me with so much love. 'I am who you truly are. Be with me and you will truly understand that all there is, is love. The rest is but a movie.' My heart exploded. I have never felt so ecstatic. The being gradually dissolved as we were served lunch on the ward. I couldn't eat the meat. I kept seeing it as our golden retriever being served up on a dish. Meat has feelings. Only veg for me.

The lessons began as I spent that month in Long Grove. I was shown the stages of existence. They were likened to the floors of a house. I was shown that the responsibilities, from those of a cleaner all the way up to a king, were a direct result of soul karma. One couldn't skip a stage. We all had to experience everything.

I was told to get ready to get on a plane, where I would fulfil my existence. It was an aeroplane where everyone got on two by two, just like on Noah's ark. 'Can I take Liz with me?' I said to the voice. 'She is not your truth in this life – you must go alone.' I could see my musical talents come to fruition as service to the world at the end of this flight, but could I give up Liz? The energy on the ward intensified. An old boy with no teeth flashed a card in front of me. It said, 'There but for the Grace of God go I.' Chaos ensued as the plane left without me. I knew that I couldn't leave Liz, and as I faced this crush on my ego an extraordinary thing happened. Everyone on the ward was running around frenetically. I felt myself turning into an enormous baby, blinking out over the whole universe. I felt myself expanding into absolute consciousness. There was nothing but this one awareness. I could not withstand this experience. It was far too powerful.

At this moment a very judgemental nurse came towards me with a tablet. I didn't like her at all. 'This will help you sleep,' she said. I was shown the life when as a Christian she had slit my tongue for 'speaking in tongues'. The mystics of that time, when suppressed, are said to have had this trademark of a slit in the front of their tongue. The following night I had an irresistible urge to sing. I woke up my friend Sue, who had cut her fringe diagonally with a pair of scissors. 'Where are we going?' she said. 'To the dining room, to sing,' I replied.

That night my favourite nurse was on, the one from the Philippines, who let me do what I liked. I began to sing and dance on the dining tables, as Sue skipped around the room, laughing. Suddenly I came to a standstill and couldn't move. 'What's wrong?' said Sue. 'Look!' I said. There were roses strewn across the floor, making a perfect pathway of petals. I followed them to the door of the dining room, travelling in slow motion. 'You're going to get out!' said the voice inside. But the door was tightly locked. Reality hit once again.

Next day, came the final lesson. Robin Day and *Question Time*. Two teams: on the one side were the more liberal members of my family, and on the other side people in my life by whom I felt constricted. A waterfall of information came through.

My father and I had experienced many lives together. Never harmoniously. I became violently angry and began punching everything in sight. The nurses were afraid of me. The voice within said, 'This is not the way.' 'But look what he's done,' I said. 'I'm sorry,' they said. Forgiveness is the only answer. I was bewildered and right about everything (so I thought). It couldn't be right, what was happening in the Government with Mrs Thatcher. In that moment, I saw the underworld of politicians using prostitutes and knocking them off in car boots, like the mafia, in the woods. 'This world's corrupt!' I exclaimed. 'You must go beyond this,' said the voice, 'This is your mission.' I saw a flash vision of an expanded mansion house that in the future would support and nourish people who were going through a similar experience to mine. It was a place where they would be understood and supported through their confusion. I began chanting with all my heart, and was then blessed with a vision of all my dearest friends coming towards me with candles, in a procession in the sky.

I got the lesson. These experiences were for me only. I should keep quiet about them. No 'pearls before swine'. I began to be obedient on the ward. I stopped giving my brand new pyjamas away. I helped in the kitchen and washed the floors. I was polite and ordinary. The doctors approved me, and one month later I was released.

The transformation of my reality

That year was a turnaround. I had undergone a genuine and lasting transformation. It enabled me to give up alcohol and drugs. I went into a recovery programme and, only six months after leaving the hospital, was cast at the Royal National Theatre in *Peer Gynt* and *The Good Person of Szechuan* – both stories about individuals looking for the meaning of life. I don't think this was a coincidence either.

I resumed my chanting and meditation practice, and became stronger in my enthusiasm and connection to spirit. It took me two years to find the courage to leave Liz – a very sad event. She has a special place in my heart today as an agent of the hands of God in my life.

In 1990, I began training in sound vibration work, and was soon beginning to run my own singing groups. The work has developed over the years in so many extraordinary ways. I have called my company 'Free The Inner Voice', as I recognize how vital it is to have a voice in this world, not only simply to sing, but also to be able to speak up for yourself and others who are vulnerable, oppressed or stigmatized in any way. I have worked in several mental health areas, with drink and drug addicts, children and teenagers, and in the business world, and I continue to do so with the general public.

In more recent years, having finally moved on from the theatre world, I find myself writing and singing my own songs, songs of the soul, in public performances throughout each year. My dream is to release my own album. In this ambition, I have been inspired by the efforts and success in 2000 of a group of long-term mental health users I was working with. Through the sound work we did together, these disadvantaged men and women were able to write their own words and music. Thirteen of their songs subsequently appeared on a CD, which was fully sponsored by an award from the Mind Millennium Grant fund. Our label is 'CARSOS' (standing for 'Creative Arts Resource for the Sanity of the Soul'). Proceeds from this album go towards empowering other mental health users back into creative reality through music and song. Like this book, the CD is entitled 'Breakthrough', because for many of us involved, that is what this successfully empowering project has been.

My journey came full circle in 2002. My friend and ally, psychiatrist Dr Larry Culliford, invited me not only to speak of my experiences (much as described here) to a meeting of psychiatrists and trainees, but also to run a voice workshop for a group of 30 psychiatrists. This took place in a Cardiff Conference Centre at the Annual Meeting of the Royal College of Psychiatrists. It is very possible that this was the same location as my own 'breakthrough' – another natural coincidence surely.

The highlight of every week for me currently is to work with recovering addicts in a renowned hospital in north London. They are so close to my heart, and surely this is a way of giving back something of what I gained through my own rocky ride to freedom.

I am also now part of a wonderful research team of psychiatrists and alternative healers who are setting up 'The Orchard Foundation'. This exciting venture is being steered to fruition by Maya Parker, a psychotherapist. The project, at the planning stage at present, is to develop a 'spiritual emergency centre'. Those involved are expecting to truly address the fine line between mystical growth experiences and mental breakdown. My involvement is to be a teacher and guide in the field of sound and music, working with the voice as an agent of healing. I believe it is possible that this foundation is connected to my vision of the mansion house from my days in the hospital so many years ago.

I conclude in saying I am now in a happy union with my beloved partner Yasia, who I met through the field of voice. She is my constant cheerleader and loving friend. My relationship with my family is also fully reconciled and restored to peace, and my father and I are now excellent friends.

The rest I let the grace of spirit reveal, because I feel sure we are all in this world together, ultimately Heavenbound!

Afterword

It has taken 12 years of deep reflection and revelation to understand the experiences that I have described in this chapter. It is as if they happened to me in that period and that I would come to appreciate their blessing in retrospect!

As I perceive it now, I received in 1989 the descent of Grace from a lineage of yogic masters. This manifested as an awakening of my kundalini energy coiled at the base of my spine. This can be compared to the Holy Spirit of the Christian tradition, or the awakened Chi of the Taoist tradition, etc. This energy is supremely intelligent and is available to all who tap into her! At the appointed time of the ripening of each individual soul, we come to a point of a balance of 'good and bad' karmas, where we start to ask the question at the soul level (after many lifetimes) 'who am I?'

I believe I have wanted to know who I was in essence since I could first speak in infanthood. Nothing could satiate my hunger more than the awakening of my inner divinity. However, I didn't know that this was what I was looking for.

Upon this almighty awakening I could no longer doubt that there is an infinite loving presence in this universe and it lives inside me and in all sentient beings, waiting to be beckoned.

I now come to fully understand that my soul has incarnated before, as the chapter suggests, in Egypt, Rome and in the time of the Vedic seers of India – a detail I didn't mention. Through experience I have realized that each soul I am unresolved with from former lives I will encounter in this one or the next. For example, in this chapter my father and I have been in a point of tension for several lifetimes. I know in my heart (and that is sufficient for me) that our soul connection is at last at peace in this life!

I refer to UFOs and Martians. I know that there are other realms, other than the Earth plane, of loving beings who help us along the way. They felt strangely familiar as they spoke to me from within, leaving me doubtless of their existence.

The intelligence of kundalini showed me all the stages of evolution, from the 'shop floor up', and that I would experience all manner of things before reaching enlightenment. The vision of the blue being shimmering in front of me was a blessed preview of the highest destination and fulfilment of my journey. I had this to look forward to! I believe the sight of my meditation master, on the video screen at the front of the bus, as appearing to merge with Holly was significant. Her surname was Lingham – the name given to the seed of Shiva (consciousness). I was to move through human relationship in the root chakra all the way up to reunion with the divine feminine (portrayed by my meditation master) rooted in the crown chakra of my subtle body. The theme of the mother continued with the symbolic death of my own mother, to the emerging of the consciousness of 'Mother Earth is weeping'.

This energy knows everything before we think we know at the level of ego. It gave me prophesy of life direction, particularly the vision of the 'spiritual emergency centre' that I was to create in the future, and a fundamental insight into the shadow of society, particularly in the area of government and the level of corruption that we seldom see in public!

I now understand that the burning heat I experienced on my skin throughout my time in hospital was the kundalini purifying every cell of my being (i.e. the purging of drugs and alcohol) and hence all the past life recall and prophesy. I received the vision that once the drama of cause and effect, or the wheel of birth and death, reaches its pinnacle, nothing remains but the bliss of divine consciousness. In this reality, time no longer exists and we are profoundly at peace. To have tapped this just for one moment in my life has left me with infinite gratitude to the lineage of great beings who have awakened this 'self knowledge' within me and all seekers of the truth through many lifetimes.

Finally, I now embrace life on life's terms, enjoying its apparent paradoxes and sudden changes. No matter how rough life becomes, I can never forget the peace of my own 'inner self'.

A Commentary on 'Heavenbound'

LARRY CULLIFORD

Larry Culliford is a consultant psychiatrist. He calls himself a 'universalist' Christian, worshipping traditionally but respecting and grateful for the truths, teachings and practices of other major faith traditions. He is a member of the Thomas Merton Society and the Scientific and Medical Network. He writes spiritually oriented self-improvement books under a pen name (see www.happinesssite.com).

> Spirituality connects the one with the whole. It links the deeply personal with the universal, and each one of us thereby with each other.

It is possible that Nikki had a single episode of textbook affective disorder in 1989, with no recurrences so far, but this would be but an impoverished interpretation of the events then and since.

The best evidence of real growth and a lasting transformation for a psychiatrist, and perhaps the most deserving of our attention, is that the experience enabled Nikki to give up alcohol and drugs. It also enabled her to get her career back on track. That she is grateful and wants to help others with addiction and mental health problems provides further evidence of her newfound maturity. Her life has new meaning and purpose. She has a humble and grateful sense of destiny and mission, with guidance and support built in through her spiritual practice. Realistic about her visionary link with the Orchard Foundation and other initiatives, she is an able and effective ambassador for spiritual care.

This is a rare, special, literate and detailed account of an episode of mental illness that can teach us much. These events occurred in 1989 when Nikki was in her late twenties. I did not encounter her until the millennial year at a musical concert, part of the 'Healing Sounds' festival in Brighton.[1] In a large Victorian church building, the remarkable singer

---

[1] I wish to make clear that at no time have I acted as psychiatrist to Nikki herself.

Chloe Goodchild led a chorus of singers and musicians, and later we the audience too, in an uplifting evening of song and chanting. I noticed the energetic and talented keyboard player, clearly the lead musician, someone with a sharp awareness of rhythm and timing, and of what everyone else was doing around her. Her role was clearly to co-ordinate and enliven the music making. Only from the programme did I know this to be Nikki Slade.

On leaving, my attention was drawn to a CD for sale. This was 'Breakthrough', by CARSOS. Intrigued by the idea that a group of mental health service users had recorded it, I bought a copy. Impressed, I contacted Nikki to find out more. When we met, I asked how she got involved with this work and heard for the first time the account of her 'breakthrough'. Always on the lookout for people whose stories are instructive and carry hope, I invited Nikki to come and talk about herself to a large group of psychiatrists and trainees. Present too was hospital chaplain Stuart Johnson.

During the discussion, the older, more traditional psychiatrists, trained in the biomedical model of disease, concentrated on the 'course of illness' and the form of Nikki's symptoms, eager to identify possible brain pathology and a diagnosis. The younger group, including the trainees, were less interested in this impersonal approach; trained in the biopsychosocial model, they were looking for predisposing and precipitating or trigger factors for Nikki's 'affective psychosis', and protective factors to explain the apparent good eventual outcome. Stuart then helpfully suggested a more spiritual interpretation.

These three types of approach are not mutually exclusive; they support each other. As I have described elsewhere (Culliford, 2002), human experience can be described according to five seamlessly and hierarchically inter-related dimensions: physical, biological, intra-personal (psychological), inter-personal (familial/sociocultural) and spiritual. The latter, in one sense the most complex, subsuming and inhabiting the other four as an integrating principle, is also the simplest, by virtue of its unity and indivisibility. Such apparent paradoxes are the stuff of spirituality. The spiritual dimension is the source of the remainder – of time, space, matter and energy, of everything – and so the hierarchical system, rather than a static pyramid, is best conceived, as circular and dynamic, a poetic and mandalic vision of wholeness.

Spirituality connects the one with the whole. It links the deeply personal with the universal, and each one of us thereby with each other. According to a nursing textbook (Murray and Zentner, 1989):

> In every human being there seems to be a spiritual dimension, a quality that
> goes beyond religious affiliation, that strives for inspiration, reverence, awe,

meaning and purpose, even in those who do not believe in God. The spiritual dimension tries to be in harmony with the universe, strives for answers about the infinite, and comes essentially into focus in times of emotional stress, physical illness, loss, bereavement and death.

We can add mental illness to this list of afflictions. To do full justice to Nikki Slade's tale, then, we need to examine it, in so far as we can, from the perspective of each of these five dimensions.

There is little to say about the physical level, except a reminder that matter and energy, the basic components of the universe, are interchangeable and manifest as the atoms and molecules from which our biological systems are formed.

Important to the story at the biological level are the brain (its anatomy and physiology) the nervous and endocrine (hormone) systems of which it is a central part, and the sense organs – those of vision and hearing in particular, which seemed to go wrong as Nikki saw and heard what others could not. Long-term use and abuse of either drugs or alcohol affect brain physiology and function, and both will have played some part in Nikki's experiences. We do not have enough information about the extent or nature of drug use or alcohol intake to go into detail, however.

Neither do we have much information about Nikki's formative psychological experiences and her inner world before the onset of symptoms, only that life seemed empty and meaningless and that she was in a stagnant relationship. A psychiatrist would want to know more about her sexual orientation and whether this or any related past experiences, including experiences with men, had led to inner conflict or turmoil. Nikki's father's attitude was important to her. Could it be that he usually accepted her friends, but not Holly because she was Nikki's first female sexual partner?

There are a number of questions a psychiatrist would ask, wanting to know things not only because they may help explain the psychological crisis, but also to prepare for important psychotherapeutic work, including family therapy, later on. Nikki's creative side and the frustration involved in low-paid, menial employment – additional potential contributing factors to her predicament as the story unfolds – need further exploration too if we are to understand things fully at the psychological and inter-personal levels.

There is less need to speculate, however, when it comes to formulating a diagnosis. Nikki has provided us with a near-textbook account of 'mania with psychosis'. She describes grandiosity of thought content, accompanied in a cyclical way by suspiciousness and persecutory ideas. She experienced visual and auditory hallucinations congruent with her thoughts, and also high levels of energy and arousal. Her emotions were labile and again consistent with her thought content. She experienced intense joy and elation at times, followed by equally intense fear, anger and sorrow – when thinking she was about to be raped, for example, about what she imagined her father had done in a past life, or when believing that her mother had died.

At the biological level, there would have been a liberal release of neurotransmitters inside Nikki's limbic system at the time. This is the circuit in the brain controlling the emotions. Powerful feelings activate the cerebral cortex, stimulating and colouring thoughts, which in turn cause feedback to the limbic system, driving the emotions to even greater excess, and so on round and round.

This cyclical crescendo of activity can only be restrained by the kind of medication Nikki was given; presumably some form of antipsychotic. The alternative, eventually, is physical exhaustion and sleep, but this might only be a brief interruption before the chaotic process continues. Another outcome, probably associated with depletion of the neurotransmitters, is that the mania is followed by loss of energy and an associated psychological depression. That is why mania and its lesser form, hypomania, are considered part of so-called bipolar affective disorder, formerly called manic depression. The two are frequently linked.

Nikki writes and speaks about her month-long ordeal with no anger or bitterness. When you speak to her, she gives credit to those who treated her forcibly under the Mental Health Act. She knows that there was no alternative at the time. Her thinking was too disordered for her to articulate what was happening, and to benefit from any sophisticated psychotherapeutic intervention. What she wanted and needed was to feel safe, respected and valued.

This attitude is entirely consistent with naturalistic research studies on psychiatric patients, conducted by means of focus groups, interviews and questionnaires. According to Mary Nathan's study (Nathan, 1997), for example, the elements of spiritual care that patients say they require include:

- An environment for purposeful activity such as creative art, structured work, enjoying nature.
- Feeling safe and secure. Being treated with respect and dignity, and allowed to develop a feeling of belonging, of being valued and trusted.
- Having time to express feelings to staff members with a sympathetic, listening ear.
- Opportunities and encouragement to make sense of and derive meaning from experiences, including illness experiences.
- Receiving permission and encouragement to develop a relationship with God or the Absolute (however the person conceives whatever is

sacred). Thus having a time, a place and privacy in which to pray and worship, receiving education in spiritual (and sometimes religious) matters, encouragement in deepening faith, and feeling universally connected and perhaps also forgiven.

The benefits described include:

- Improved self-control, self-esteem and confidence.
- Recovery is facilitated, both by promoting the healthy grieving of loss and through maximizing personal potential.
- Relationships are improved – with self, others and with God or the Absolute.
- A sense of meaning develops, resulting in renewed hope and peace of mind, enabling people to accept and live with their problems.

So, we can ask, where does meaning reside within the strange experiences that Nikki has so clearly described?

According to a paper by Rosemarie McCabe and her co-workers (McCabe et al., 2002): 'Patients repeatedly attempted to talk about the content of their psychotic symptoms in the out-patient setting.' 'This,' they said, 'was a source of noticeable interactional tension and difficulty.'

Psychiatrists are still taught to take more notice of the form of a person's illness, and to treat the symptoms, than to help the person find meaning in them. Such is the state of our materialist culture, that many feel discouraged from discovering the spiritual dimension in their own lives, and therefore shy away from it in others, especially their patients. In rehabilitation psychiatry, however, we have had to teach ourselves how to redress this imbalance.

To ignore the spiritual dimension is to ignore important resources: those within the person providing energy and enthusiasm, motivation and hope; and those which are external, supplied through that person's faith tradition and/or spiritual support network. It is important to distinguish spirituality, which is essentially unifying, from religion, which may be divisive; and to distinguish faith, which is deep-seated, personal and incontrovertible, from beliefs, which are open to question and doubt. The first step, we have found, is to ask patients what helps to sustain them. Most will then reveal something of their spiritual life.

Nikki tells us little of her initial religious upbringing and faith tradition. Raised in England, the main influence is likely to have been Christian, an idea supported by her calling repetitively on 'Jesus Christ our Lord' when in fear. As her story begins, she has, however, embarked on a spiritual path involving a female master or teacher, sacred yoga, meditation and chanting. She calls it now 'A universal path of love'. This might have represented another major challenge to her family and friends, as Nikki's lifestyle and values began to change away from theirs.

Yoga and chanting, like meditation, serve a purpose (Whiteside, 2003). Put simply, it is to enable us each separately to improve our experience of our existing connection with the universal whole, and also thereby with each other. To go full on, especially unguided, into the spiritual experience carries risks, especially the risk of the kind of disjunction from everyday normality that we refer to as 'psychosis'. For most people, then, especially those from a materialist, evidence-based, science-orientated culture, an ideal spiritual quest proceeds at a slow and gradual pace. It involves a great deal of unlearning and re-evaluating of pre-conditioned assumptions. And it often involves leaving others in your peer group behind until you have made sufficient progress to re-engage with them and contribute helpfully to their education. Otherwise both intra- and inter-personal conflicts occur readily.

To put it briefly, meditation can assist us to make progress through what James Fowler described as the six stages of faith (Fowler, 1980). The first two concern pre-adolescence, by which time most people will have entered Stage Three. The moment you realize that, at the deepest level, you are personally at odds with your culture, and with it the values, assumptions and beliefs of your family, teachers and those around you; you leave behind the security afforded by belonging to a group. You leave the safe but nevertheless incomplete position of Stage Three and enter the more difficult terrain of Stage Four. If the dissonance is great and the realization is abrupt, a psychological crisis with symptoms of psychosis can easily happen.

Psychiatrists do well to know about this. Our understanding has moved on from when Carl Jung indicated that sufferers of schizophrenia had experiences with universally resonant and relevant content (Fordham, 1966). We have progressed too from RD Laing's descriptions of personal growth through psychotic experience (Laing, 1967). We are ready to begin distinguishing the destructive from the creative, the breakdown from the breakthrough. As well as minimizing the hurt and harm of the former, we are ready to learn effective means of promoting the latter. We may even be able to assist in transforming breakdowns into breakthroughs. We should be confident and hopeful, but our wisdom on this is significantly incomplete still.

The importance of Nikki's account is in showing us that the move into Stage Four can rapidly, if painfully and confusingly, precede a continuation into the more satisfactory position of Stage Five, the universalist position.

Beyond uncertainty, Stage Five is the position of wisdom, compassion and faith. It is the non-partisan, non-dualist position, wherein an individual feels him or herself to be allied spontaneously with all people, with all beings and all creation. Reaching Stage Five, it is said, is like coming home.[2] The life of the person who has arrived here is a blessing to all. It is not the end of pain, because to identify compassionately with others in their suffering is to feel their pain as your own. However, resistance to the experience of painful emotions is over. The natural processes of psychological healing are allowed to flow unhindered towards resolution, resulting in personal growth and maturity. When equanimity is restored, it leaves you free to think clearly then speak and act wisely (or wisely refrain from speaking or acting) for the benefit of all concerned.

There are signs that Nikki was making a transition through Stage Four and into Stage Five. This, at least, is one way of making sense of what occurred. In doing so, it is also necessary to postulate that she was somehow in direct contact with the spiritual realm or dimension that is somehow beyond life and death. The link came abruptly and decisively when she began meditation and chanting. 'Three days into the practice, something happened,' she said. 'I felt warmth in my heart, and a friendliness that I automatically wanted to share.' She felt 'very connected' to the radio, and grew concerned about the ozone layer. She saw a resemblance between a human and a creature from the ape kingdom. A beautiful sunset became an ecstatic extension of her body.

Nikki's account continues, 'The duality of my perception dissolved and I felt absolutely connected to every tree, bird, dog, lake, person, in fact to Nature in her entirety.' Later, she adds, 'My awareness was timeless' and she boards a 'heavenbound' train. On another occasion she says, 'It occurred to me for a split second that I had been more than, and would again be more than, only Nikki Slade.' We could call this Nikki getting in touch with her soul. But these experiences quickly brought problems.

The first forceful glimpse of the spiritual seems to have highlighted pre-existing difficulties in Nikki's life that required attention. Her problem relationship with Liz is centre stage at the beginning, introducing material about her friendship with Holly and friction with her father in the form of 'past-life' experiences. Whether you think of these as true or the product of creative, dreamlike imagination, their effect on Nikki was significant. They stirred up powerful, apparently truthful, emotions of joy and love as well as suspicion and fear.

Nikki describes trying to go on with her commitments regarding social activities and the fashion show, but her symptoms grew stronger. A way of understanding this is to say that her personal ego was at odds with her spiritual self, which seemed alien and was therefore split off. This projected aspect of her greater self communicated with her through voices,

---

[2] Stage Six, according to Fowler, is one of almost superhuman faith and ability, the realm of martyrs and saints.

which Nikki identified as those of extraterrestrials, warning, for example, against the use of drugs as spiritually deadening agents. Her spiritual self (or 'wisdom mind') communicated with her, too, through meaningful coincidences (referred to by Jung as 'synchronicities'), also through archetypes and symbols such as the Egyptian characters, a magical cat, a biblical storm, Shiva's lingam, a royal red carpet, golden chariots, the angelic guardian, Mother Earth, Caesar and the Romans, an old woman, a burning bodily heat and 'a radiant being in electric blue robes, with jet black hair and charcoal eyes, dripping with dew'.

The spiritual dimension is mediated more concretely through the image of Nikki's teacher, who is real and who we may assume to have reached an advanced Stage Five, or even Stage Six, in terms of faith development. This master is therefore a genuine guide and source of inspiration. The significance of the crown chakra, access to which is the pinnacle of kundalini yoga, is that it implies spiritual fulfilment. The reference to Holly's merging with the master arguably signifies the transformation of earthbound, erotic and possessive love to a more mature, selfless and universal form. This is universal, spiritual love.

Nikki's task, as she went through a fast-forward Stage Four, was to effect a reunification of the split in her psyche revealed by these events, a reconciliation of all conflict in her mind – between herself and her 'past-life' father, between earth and heaven, West and East, past and present, present and future, between holding on to that which she valued and loved and letting it go – because there was no real choice. 'I couldn't accept death as a reality that all of us face,' she said. 'Mother Earth is weeping, and we must act now ... The force within me was so strong that I was afraid ... I knew that I couldn't leave Liz.'

The inner struggle is typified by the quiz game. Nikki describes it as 'Two teams: on the one side were the more liberal members of my family, and on the other people in my life by whom I felt constricted.' But Nikki's spiritual connectedness seems to have pulled her through. She discovered the answer within the higher self that she has, with the help of her teacher, yoga, chanting and meditation, come to trust.

This is how it goes. Using Nikki's words: 'We all had (have) universal bliss within us.' 'I was shown the stages of existence. They were likened to the floors of a house. One couldn't skip a stage. We all had to experience everything.' 'A burning in my body began from head to toe ... This was no ordinary heat. I have come to understand that this was spiritual energy doing its work, cleansing the impressions of lifetimes.' And, using the words of her voices: 'Your father has saved you ... He is a good man.' 'Forgiveness is the only answer.' 'All there is, is love, Nikki. When you see this, you will understand that none of this is real.' 'I am who you truly are. Be with me and you will truly understand that all there is, is love.'

As Nikki entered Stage Five, a new insight was dawning. 'An unbelievable compassion arose within me. I saw everyone I'd ever known and all I felt was love. All battles were over.' It enabled her to do what had to be done, to let go of the wish and desire to remain in control against the inevitable. 'I stopped resisting.' 'Finally, I surrendered.' And then it was like a rebirth: 'I felt myself turning into an enormous baby, blinking out over the whole universe. I felt myself expanding into absolute consciousness. There was nothing but this one awareness.'

How are we to make sense of this in terms of everyday psychology? There is a way. We can do so in terms of attachment and loss.

The earthbound ego is primarily attached to itself, to existence, to life. It feels threatened by death, of course, and also by the infinite, in which it fears itself insignificant. Grandiose egocentricity is its defence, but the price of this is to feel threatened with persecution and punishment, to experience strong emotions associated with threat, especially fear and anxiety. Defiance of threat and resistance against the effects of loss, especially if denial is involved, are associated with the emotion of anger. When, however, the inevitability of loss can no longer be ignored, the first phase of acceptance brings sadness, often a precursor of healing and growth. These three distressing emotions – fear, anger and sadness – were prominent in Nikki's account of her transformative experiences. The everyday ego-mind was painfully lost and had to be relinquished, before a new and greater, wiser, more compassionate and universal self could be reborn in its place (Whiteside, 2001).

How do we know that this transformation was genuine and likely to be lasting? The best evidence comes from meeting Nikki herself, seeing her perform as a musician, leading a workshop or simply relaxing in the company of her new partner, Yasia. She is vibrant and happy, a true inspiration to those she works with and those she meets.

References

Culliford L (2002) Spiritual care and psychiatric treatment: an introduction. Advances in Psychiatric Treatment 8: 249–261.

Fordham F (1966) An Introduction to Jung's Psychology, 3rd edn. Harmondsworth: Penguin.

Fowler J (1980) Stages of Faith: the psychology of human development and quest for meaning. London: HarperCollins.

Laing RD (1967) The Politics of Experience and the Bird of Paradise. Harmondsworth: Penguin.

McCabe R, Heath C, Burns T and Priebe S (2002) Engagement of patients with psychosis in the consultation: conversation analytic study. British Medical Journal 325: 1148–1151.

Murray RB and Zentner JP (1989) Nursing Concepts for Health Promotion. London: Prentice Hall.

Nathan MM (1997) A study of spiritual care in mental health practice: patients' and nurses' perceptions. MSc thesis, Middlesex University, Enfield.

Whiteside P (2001) Happiness: the 30-day guide. London: Rider Books.

CHAPTER 13

Broken Chains

SUE HOLT

Sue Holt has spent a lot of time since 1997 in and out of a psychiatric hospital.

> At first I was very ashamed and broken by my experience, both about being ill and my inability to cope, and the reactions of those around me. Over time I saw my distress in a different light to those around me. I gained hope, faith and a new inner strength. I tried hard to convince others to see it my way and eventually realized they were incapable of seeing it as I did. It was my experience. This gave me the confidence to further accept my experience as I believed it, while accepting that others have their own perceptions of me.
>
> At the moment I live each day with a quiet sense of wonder that surprises and amazes me. I am doing an art course at college, I go to a local user group, and help publish and distribute a newsletter. Within the last year I have become a member of a user/carer training team, which provides training to other users, carers and professionals.

Charting the background

I have had ten major psychotic episodes, but I am aware that I have also had minor ones, which have not needed hospital care. I was also sexually abused as a child.

I am diagnosed as having manic depression/bipolar disorder. For me this means so many things. First, that I have mood swings, which go from suicidal to psychotic, and second, that I need medication at this present moment to help me regulate the mood swings. All of this classes me as having experienced madness and I am aware it also leaves the door open for that to potentially reoccur in the future.

When I was first diagnosed it meant much more to me. I thought I could no longer have a worthwhile place in society. I was also very aware of society's views of the mentally ill and madness, and at first I did not want anything to do with other people who were mentally ill or with mental health services. I thought I *was* my label. I had to deal with a lot of stigma within myself, about my feelings towards me. I was incredibly ashamed and frightened of what the future held and I was told, over and over again, that I was disabled. Now I realize I do have a mental illness and if I become too complacent or do too much, or do anything particularly stressful, that it will take its toll on me.

The first flush of madness

My first episode occurred just after giving birth to my son in 1990. I believe it represented my special way of coping with life at that time. I was ill-prepared to be a mother – emotionally, physically, spiritually or mentally. The trauma of my son's birth reconnected me to my past, especially to memories of being abused by my stepfather. The birth was so traumatic but, apart from pushing, I played very little part in it. I actually felt tortured. The birth was very complicated; my son had the umbilical cord wrapped around his neck, and forceps and a vacuum were used to remove him. This was one of my worst nightmares, as one of my sisters has cerebral palsy and I had trained in the care of people with learning disabilities, so I was aware that problematic births could lead to brain injury.

So, I escaped from all this pain into a world of beauty. I believed my son was Jesus Christ. I really don't know how it happened, as at that time I wasn't religious in any way, shape or form. I just knew! I remember singing carols from my childhood – like 'Little Drummer Boy' and 'Little Donkey' – and I felt very festive, although my son was born in October. In my eyes the world had now become a safe place to be. Colours were vivid. It felt good to be alive. However, I was told no such world existed here on Earth.

Stolen experiences

The first person to say this was my health visitor. I told her that I had gone for a walk at 10pm and it was like teatime, and that it was peaceful and people were out walking with their children. She said that was ridiculous as no one would be out at that time with their children. On reflection, I believe that my feelings/thoughts/experiences were stolen from me, as they were not recognized as being real and important to me at that moment in time. Everyone stole these experiences, from my health visitor, to my GP, to my husband, to my psychiatrist. The stealing was devastating, as I believed it was so real, and it led to so much confusion for me and resulted in my becoming very depressed. You don't know what to believe when your mind and senses and thoughts are telling you one thing and people around you are saying, 'Well actually it's not true'. However, apart from the time when I was really suicidal, all my experiences were good, and I so wanted them to be real. But once again people didn't understand that and they just talked about 'denial' and 'lack of insight'.

I remember an old lady who said that I was an angel, 'a real live angel'. Oh how wonderful that made me feel. I wasn't going to argue with her. If she thought I was an angel it made us both happy, at least for that moment in time. However, a nurse said, 'Oh no, it's only Sue'. It is hard to make others understand, but for a couple of minutes, that old lady and I shared something magical, but it was spoiled. I look back and think, 'Well OK, I was "an angel" for that moment for her. Although it ended we did connect for a brief time.'

That first episode left me feeling very much abused and emotionally scared. I had talked about my childhood while in hospital, but unfortunately for me this was seen as having little importance to my current 'mental health state'.

The experience of psychosis

During one time when I was psychotic I *knew* I was being reborn spiritually. However, my spirit was very much diminished. One thing that stood out was the sense that there was no hope – there was no purpose to my life. I was plodding along. I lacked energy and motivation and felt lifeless. I was dead, empty: I was just an empty shell. I was devoid of emotions except hate, fear, resentment, and lots and lots of anger. Anger was my fuel. I didn't think beyond what was on TV or what to have for tea. I did not challenge or question. Instead, I accepted everything and then went away and muttered under my breath.

At the time of my 'spiritual rebirth' I was lying on the bed and I could 'feel' the very centre of myself. It was a tight knot inside of me: a hard lump. However, it started unravelling from the outside, in a spiral, going round and round, and I could feel it within me. It was very painful, but I was aware that I needed to go through this pain, as it was the right thing to do. I started screaming. I needed to scream. I needed to connect with my pain. My spirit knew that.

Early on, God had begun talking to me. I say 'God' because there is a part of me that would really like to believe that it was God, as it really improves my self-esteem to think that. I am also aware that it could be my subconscious or a whole host of things. However, I am now quite comfortable believing it is God. At first it was a real battle to really trust this inner voice, as I was having conflicting messages from those around me regarding what God was saying. Also I didn't trust God 100 per cent, as I believed He had let me down when I was a child. However, I have now got to the point where I trust my inner voice even if those around me are telling me otherwise. As my confidence in God grew, my spirit within me began to grow too.

The nursing staff told me not to scream, which caused a lot of frustration for me. I told them I was in pain but that it was OK. I needed to go through this pain. However, I was told I was upsetting the other patients and they offered me medication. I felt as though my experience was being questioned, and that my knowledge of myself and what I needed at that point did not count. The staff members were the experts – they knew best. I was also confused as to what was the truth. Was it their truth or my truth?

Believing and doubting

I had numerous battles with Satan and evil spirits, and believed I was battling for my soul. My awareness of this 'spiritual struggle' came on suddenly, but I was too frightened to talk about it. I was also too frightened of Satan's power, but once I read Job I realized God allows Satan only so much power. All of this had a big impact on my life. I have asked myself, 'Is there really any such thing as an ordinary life?' OK, I know I was not spiritual before all of this happened, but I knew that I was on the wrong road and I needed to get off it. I think that such experiences are different for different people; some come slowly and some, like me, come suddenly.

When I am admitted to hospital I am very aware of the highly charged atmosphere in the building. I feel it is in the air. I feel it in the furniture. I feel it everywhere. One day I knew I could clean up the atmosphere. I opened the window and put out my face (as the window wouldn't open fully) and I opened my mouth. I could feel the badness moving through me and out of my mouth. As my breath touched the outside air I believed that it became clean energy.

Once, I believed that God had told me to go to Heaven, and he sent a UFO to take me there. On reflection, I think that the significance of the UFO involved the way my mind made use of a circular dining table. At that time, I didn't completely trust God so I dithered a while before I went. By the time I got there (Heaven) the Devil had arrived before me and Heaven was ruined, all black and dirty. I remember thinking that I had died to see this and it was all ruined. I felt cheated and had a real fear of God taking me to Heaven before I was ready. I was beginning to find a real life and I didn't want to die. However, God reminded me that I wasn't really dead and I felt OK. Then God told me that if I trusted Him, and believed in Him, it would be OK next time. So I got back on my UFO to go back. At this point I was asked to move. My UFO was a dining room table, which the staff needed to set for tea.

It was all very complicated, to say the least. I would be halfway to Heaven when someone would nudge me and I would be back in the ward, semi-aware; but also more aware that Heaven is just around the corner. And so I would set off again. I never did get a chance to find out what Heaven was like on that day.

Throughout all of these experiences most of my thoughts and feelings were religious, which was all totally new to me. I became a Christian and this gave me hope, which I didn't have before. However, those around me did not take my faith very seriously. Even though I became a Christian I did not totally trust God, due partly, I believe, to my abusive background. I felt He had failed me. I tested God more than once but I also believe I too was tested. I have tried to find words to explain 'how' I was 'tested' and I am still unsure of my answer. I believed my faith in God was being tested on numerous occasions. It was as if He would suggest that I did something, which would be OK as He was watching over me. Would I really trust Him? One of the stupidest things I did was take my hands off the steering wheel, as I was convinced He would steer the car. Part of me believed that He was 'there for me', as I never crashed! On reflection, that really was crazy.

Another time – the only time I begged to go into hospital, as I was suicidal – God promised me I would see the hospital in a whole new light. Well I arrived and in the non-smoking room I found shelves of Christian books and Bibles. I spent a month talking to God and reading.

Breaking down and breaking up

I believe my 'breakdowns' have been exactly that: breakdowns! I grew up with a distorted perception of the world. My thoughts about myself were very negative. I so much wanted to see myself as others saw me. I believe every time I have 'broken down' and become psychotic, something powerful happened. If handled correctly this can lead to regrowth, much like cutting back a shrub. However, what happened in reality is that my growth spurt was stopped in mid-flow. The whole thing was very frustrating. I knew if I carried on doing certain things I would discover more about myself and would begin to heal. I knew that I reconnected with my past at these times and relived issues that I was unable to confront 'face to face', as they were too painful. In my psychotic state it was easier, as there was a distance in my mind, but the staff team did not accept this. I remember I was reading Revelations from the Bible on the ward and I read out Chapter 12. It made perfect sense to me. It was about my life and it comforted me. However, when I told one of the nurses she said that although she could see how I made the connection, her pastor had recently been going through Revelations and said that they were very difficult to interpret. This made me doubt what I had read and I also doubted the feelings that had been aroused when I had read it. However, today I still read that piece and it comforts me.

I believe that when people are in psychosis there is a need for hospitalization. I certainly needed a safe place and often I needed medication, but I question the levels that are given. For me, a 'safe place' would be somewhere where I would be listened to, even if those around me didn't share my views a place that I could be freer to come through the psychosis, without such high doses of antipsychotic drugs. This would be a place where the ratio of nurses to patients would be much higher than it was in my experience.

I believe that psychosis is a chance for fundamental change, which is being stopped by the psychiatric system in the name of caring. As I have said, I have had ten major episodes of psychosis, and each one has been different for me and each one has taught me something new about myself. Some of these things were good and obviously others were not. Over time I have also learned to disregard what others say about my experience. They are just observers – not actual participants. Despite being on the sidelines of my life they are very willing to tell me what I experience.

I believe that through my various psychotic episodes I have undergone a major identity crisis. I didn't know who I was. People around me were unhelpful in their willingness to tell me who I was. For example I was told that I was 'disabled', and that I was a 'difficult' patient. I was held down and injected on numerous occasions and kept in seclusion for a while. The one positive thing I was told was that if I could do something I would – if I couldn't then I wouldn't.

Self-knowledge

I still don't really know who I am in any absolute sense. I am Sue Holt. I am a wife and a mother. But that is also about my husband and my son. That's just a part of me. Like my illness, I am a complex person. I used to think I was boring, but no longer. In reality I really don't know who I am.

I change each day, sometimes each minute. Life can make me cry one minute and laugh the next. I may read a book one day and not be able to stomach it the next. I am so topsy-turvy. Parts of me are a reflection of those around me – my family, my parents and my friends. But also there is a 'me' trying to climb out, to express myself in whatever way I can, but yet I am a vessel for the Spirit that is growing within me, which urges me to push the boundaries around me and take risks.

I do know where I have been. I know I have great courage and conviction and I know that has grown out of my experience. I know I have an increased spiritual awareness. I know my 'mental illness' came about through inner pain, loss, shame, despair and lack of spirit, but I also know that the psychiatric system does not take these into consideration. These areas need more consideration than they are getting at the moment from the services. I often wonder why there is such fear about looking at these areas in psychiatry.

When I was psychotic I was aware of what I was doing. However, others around me weren't, and were so fearful of my actions that their reactions were based on their fears and perceptions, rather than on 'me'. I was rarely asked what it was I was doing. However, I am now aware that I found it difficult to communicate to those around me, as they were not looking at the world through my eyes. However, this is only to be expected. I often ask, 'So I don't think like you? Were you brought up exactly like me? Have you shared my experiences? No, therefore it is obvious that your thoughts will be different, but mine are considered odd.'

I believe that by writing this I may help someone, somewhere, who is struggling with their experiences. Certainly it is helping me. Being asked to do this was a huge buzz. When I first had that thought, my reaction was 'You're crazy, you're getting high'. Then I wondered, 'Is that my real thought or has it been imposed on me by the system and by my past experiences of the world and myself?' It's OK to think small. It's like believing that everything happens for a reason. Well I didn't believe that once but I do now, so there will be a reason for all this. Everything connects somehow.

Looking back on my early bouts of madness, I was frightened by the experience itself, and the psychiatric system and its power. I am no longer frightened of the 'psychotic experience' itself but rather the implications – the loss of my freedom, the loss of my dignity, the power and control exercised by my 'carers'.

For me, psychosis has been a challenge; something I was ill-prepared for or was inadequately helped to deal with. However, that challenge has helped to remould and rejuvenate me. Today I know I am alive because of my experience, whereas before I was just an automaton going through life.

For me I feel my psychotic history has been a natural healing process.

Broken Chains

I thought I knew you Lord
But today you showed me, how wrong I was.
I was sitting in a very deep pit
Deep and dark with slippery sides
And the more I attempted
To climb
Those walls
The more I became covered
In sticky secretions
Which further hampered my movements.

I called out to you for mercy
And you answered my call
You came to my assistance
And offered me new life
You sat on the edge of the pit
With your hand out stretched to me
Forgive me Lord
For not answering your call.

I continued to struggle
In the pit of despair
Becoming more and more entrenched
In the filth that was there.
Again and again I prayed
For an end to the pain
But yet I ignored
You and your gift of love.

You have so much compassion
You could not bear to witness
My pain.
So my Lord
You leapt into the darkness
Alongside me
To comfort me and to relieve me
Of some of my anguish
To fight some of my demons
On my behalf.

Today, Lord
You whispered gently
In my mind.
You chastised me
Sweetly.
You told me you could no longer stay
With me
In my pit.
It was time to move on
Together.

You took my hand in yours
And said trust me
With all your heart.
With your awesome power
You filled my pit with radiant light
And turned it on to its side
Lord you led me out
By your side.

We walked through a green field
And came to a rusty gate
Barred by chains and locks
And barbed wire.
At one word from you
The bolts slid away
And the chains were broken in two.
As we stepped through the gate
It immediately closed
Behind us
And new signs appeared
Saying keep out
Trespassers will be shot.

You led me through
A spring meadow
Full of fresh green growth
And daffodils
Gently swaying in the breeze
You led me to a wooden bench
Looking out at a vast lake
You told me to rest
And be at peace at last.

CHAPTER 14

Spirituality, Madness and the Man Who Lost a Thousand Masks

GARY PLATZ

Gary Platz was born in Cooroy in southeast Queensland in 1952 and spent his childhood on a dairy farm near a town called Kenilworth.

> After school I moved to New Zealand, to avoid being drafted to Vietnam in the Australian army, and have lived there most of the time since. I married in 1979 and started a window-cleaning business, which I did until I developed 'mental illness'. After a three-year period of not working I started doing part-time volunteering, running some groups for fellow consumers, then doing support work and running a day programme centre. Now I am a director of a consumer consulting company, Case Consulting Ltd, and consumer advisor for Wellink Trust, a non-governmental organization that works in the community, alongside people who experience mental illness. I am involved in several consumer networks and organizations, and consider myself a writer and performing poet.

The man who lost a thousand masks

The man was a master builder
He built a thousand walls
He was an artist
Painted a face for every occasion

The man was an entrepreneur
Only paying when his price was right
He was an athlete
It was his performance that kept him in awe

The man was a pilot
Flying high hoping never to land
He was a truck driver
Always moving his load from one place to the next

The man was a church tower sniper
Shooting down what he could not bear to see
He was an undertaker
Forever burying things at great cost

Now he's the man who lost a thousand masks
Sitting by the window
He's a researcher
Gazing, pondering over why
It had to take insanity to do it

Spirituality, madness and recovery

For me spirituality wasn't a factor in recovery from madness towards some form of sanity. Rather, madness was essential in the recovery process from a spiritual crisis. To explain, I need to define the meanings of spirituality and madness as well as giving some of the context of my life story.

Spirituality

Spirituality is the ownership of love, justice, wisdom and power that is given from a source that is not of the physical. The vital ingredients are:

- Sense of self and a relationship with something of the spirit outside of self.
- The motivating energy one feels from the given forces of love, wisdom, justice and power.
- The desire to use those forces harmoniously.

Madness

Some of the words dictionaries use to define madness are: aberration, craziness, delusion, dementia, derangement, insanity, lunacy, mania, mental illness, psychopathy and psychosis.

I would *now* define my madness as the forced unleashing of the body's creative power, causing me to become aware of the vital importance of things I had ignored far too long. This understanding has come with hindsight. There was a time I was absolutely certain that it was God's Holy Spirit anointing me as Jesus Christ.

Recovery

Recovery involves making sense of, and integrating, my 'psychotic' experiences with my personal environment, and social and cultural structures, in such a way as to work towards my life of choice.

My context – my story

I shall flesh out two major experiences in my life and, with the benefit of hindsight and a major amount of writing and much personal work on myself, will try to explain what I mean by the statement: 'My madness was essential in the recovery process from a spiritual crisis.'

My entry into the mental health system happened when in my late thirties. My first experiences of *mental illness* was hearing abusive and secretive voices and having disturbing thoughts, memories and images about my past.

Whispering faces, fingers pointing straight and long, one pair of lying eyes.

This was very surprising and frightening for me, as I was not accustomed to thinking of my past and did not remember much of my childhood.

Pictures, silent, without emotion,
Forced through swollen and rusting seams of some long forgotten black box,
Flooding my consciousness.
School classrooms, his one hand on my shoulder the other reaching down
Dark storerooms, scout camps late at night
Like an obedient dog I follow
Voices wailing
Like wind through the trees

These words and images brought up a cold fury and murderous thoughts. This caused an enormous internal conflict. I had for 15 years been what would be considered a very religious man and these thoughts were in total conflict with everything I believed in. This conflict was so great I was unable to function any more. I couldn't work. I lost my business and ended up on an invalid's benefit. Everything that I had thought and every value I had held for so long became foreign, indeed *alien*, to me. For years I identified as one of Jehovah's Witnesses, with all of its associated values. I was a married man with young children and carried that story. I had my own business and all the stuff that goes with that. There seemed to be nothing of me left.

In time, through memories returning and a reconnection with my family of origin, I found out that as a child I had been sexually abused over a long period of time. So, I had counselling and worked on abuse issues, and in due course things started going quite well. Then they started going very well and then before I knew it they were going so well that I became Jesus Christ. After that I just became someone with a 'mental illness', a chronic one, with a frightening name. That is when I became really labelled.

Who am I to say who I am
When I'm told my brain isn't right
And people give it names
Which take away mine
Yes this stigma acid eats my soul

I talk of my madness being essential in the recovery process from a spiritual crisis. I also speak of being what would be considered very religious. So what was the spiritual crisis and how did madness figure in the recovery process?

One of the problems with sexual abuse and suppression of memories is that you are left with the aftermath (emotional and spiritual consequences) but you are not conscious of any cause. With a conscious cause it could have been: *I feel wrong, I feel weak, I feel less, I find it hard to trust* because of being abused.

Without any conscious cause it's simply: I am wrong, I am weak, I am less, I don't trust. This is where the spiritual crisis comes in.

- How could I ever have a sense of ownership of love, wisdom, justice and power that was given from a source not of the physical?
- How could I have a healthy relationship with something of the spirit outside of self?
- How could I have a healthy sense of self?
- How could I have any of those things when what I knew was: I am wrong, I am weak, I am less, I don't trust.

Beauty she was my friend
Till the vampire my neck

At an early age I compensated by using drugs heavily.

Rainbows at right angles, Sun flakes settling on the lawn

Pink Floyd did that to me wayback then, though the music was only partly responsible.

She came back to me for a while
Till the poisonous nights caught up

I stopped taking drugs.

The trouble was that rainbows just became things that dragged
away the clouds
Only pull out another blue day.

I then became involved in religion.

Beauty was at my side
When I saw the vision of glowing light

I could not keep it up.

That faded as my dark hole deepened

My spiritual crisis stayed with me no matter how hard I worked. I didn't know it was a spiritual crisis I didn't even know I was working hard. I did know I *was* wrong, I *was* weak, I *was* less and I *didn't trust*.

Recovery journey from spiritual crisis

For many years, through study of the Bible and endeavouring to put into practice what I learned, I had developed strong religious views that, for me, answered a lot of external questions about the state of the world, the future of mankind. I developed a belief in God. All of this was very important for me, as I had always despaired about what was going on in the world and the destruction of nature, etc. Through this time I also was able to free myself of substance dependency, get married and have a family. There was a problem, though, which was never addressed: maladaptive schemas that filtered all my thinking (I *am* less, I *am* wrong, I *am* weak, I *don't trust*). Many people think some of these schemas are implicit in the religious framework of the Bible and I guess some of them are, when comparing myself to a perfect spiritual being. The problem was I believed these things in comparison to everyone else. No matter how hard I tried I could not really trust any god-like figure.

'Madness' started for me very subtly. In fact it didn't start with 'madness' at all, but with a psychological safety net. I am sure this net saved my life many times, catching me when I fell. One day I was sitting in my work van having lunch when I began thinking about a dog I had when I was a child. This was very unusual for me, as I remembered very little of my childhood and seldom thought about what I did remember. I then started writing a story about 'Mike'. (Writing was something I didn't do.) Over the next few weeks I wrote every spare moment I could. I started staying awake at night to write. I found it difficult to work because all I wanted to do was write. I didn't realize it at the time, but I was creating a safe place to retreat to when I needed.

I wrote about the farm:

A morning bowl of cornflakes on the veranda steps
At the bottom of the gentle ridge moments of green and gold
When the early sun reaches into the river fog and finds the silky oak trees.
Another breakfast before running across the paddocks down to the school bus stop.

I wrote about the river:

> Crouching chin deep at the bottom end of a shady pool,
> Breathless as two platypuses play in the evening light,
> The small ripples disappearing under river bank ferns.

I wrote about the mountains:

> Timber clad Wall-i mountain the corner stone of the two valleys
> Up there the giant Morten Bay fig trees are king.

I wrote about the wildlife:

> I felt the warm flinch as I reached under my bed and took hold of the bat.
> They always sleep there hanging upside down from the wire weave when I
> leave the window open.

I wrote about talking to my dog, Mike:

> Mike, the teacher took me out in front of the class and hit me on the arse
> with the blackboard ruler today. Rosser and Madden were laughing because
> they could see tears in my eyes when I sat back down.

Not long after I started writing I began developing 'symptoms'. Within a couple of months I was in a psychiatric ward for the first time, *clinging to paper and pen*.

One night on the ward I lost my pen. I really panicked and needed to get out. I ran to the ward doors, which were firmly bolted. I grabbed the handles, gave a great bellow and pulled. The doors broke top and bottom and I ran kicking and screaming all the way.

> Voices, trapped, screaming
> Splitting my head
> Explosions, orange and red
> Doors splitting
> Corridor windows blurred
> Stars, buildings pulsing
> Flying rage faster than the wind

When I later returned, still extremely agitated, I was isolated and medicated. This did little to calm the inner turmoil. I demanded pen and paper, then sat and wrote.

> The smell of damp grass, the feel of dew under running feet as I head
> towards the milking sheds, afraid of missing the morning toast. Knowing
> Mike would be sitting waiting to eat my crusts.

I calmed and went to sleep.

This compulsion to write about my childhood was a major strategy my psyche was using to force me to address my spiritual crisis. I was forced to think of and remember my childhood. In time I wrote about my childhood abuse. I looked at why, instead of just the 'I am'. It was a powerfully disturbing and dynamic process.

Moments in wreckage and recreation.

Over time I began to know that I needed to change my view of myself. This was the essence of my spiritual crisis, a crisis that was crippling me. This brings me to another major experience: the 'psychotic' experience of being Jesus Christ – the Prince of Peace. There are many aspects to a psychotic experience: here I deal with some that I have understood and integrated.

The road to resolution

Briefly, as I wrote earlier, I began to feel better; memories and the extreme feelings began to settle down. I was able to do a few more things. But then I started to feel *really* good. I thought it was Jehovah's Holy Spirit surging through me then, but now I know it was adrenaline rushes. They were so strong that I didn't feel as though my feet were touching the ground. I wasn't sleeping. I was seeing 'visions'. I was doing rituals. I took my children out of school. Everybody who came and talked to me got caught up with my 'delusion'. This went on for a long time, until finally my partner came out of the 'spell' and had to get me committed under the Mental Health Act. To this very day I have a feeling of knowing I am Jesus Christ. It is a dichotomy. I feel I am Gary Platz, citizen. I feel I am Jesus Christ. I know for certain that I am not. When you have an experience powerful enough you don't lose the feeling very easily.

To explain one way that this 'experience of madness' has worked towards curing my spiritual crisis, is to describe a psychodrama.[1] I once did. In this drama I wanted to explore two extremes of being I have experienced. One extreme was being Jesus Christ. The other was being the most impotent, powerless breathing being imaginable. (After being Jesus Christ I had a series of depressive and manic 'psychotic' experiences. These experiences were accompanied by different voices, which I haven't gone into in this writing.)

In the drama, I set myself up (standing on a chair) as me being Jesus Christ at one side of the stage area, and set someone else as me lying on

---

[1] In psychodrama, you choose people to play characters, either people or things outside of you or parts of you (mostly conflicting parts). You interact with these parts by being yourself and then being the character you have interacted with and responded to (role reversal).

the floor on the opposite side of the stage. I had God sitting off in one corner. Standing in the middle, slightly to the back of the stage, were people I wanted to connect with/have a relationship with/trust and feel trusted.

It became apparent very early on in the drama that the period of time I was concerned with was the conflicted time when I still really wanted to be Jesus Christ, because it felt good. (I had to feel good to do things and being Jesus Christ is not a thing you let go of lightly.) I also wanted to be just Gary Platz. It became very clear that the reason I wanted to stop being Jesus Christ was because actually *being* Jesus Christ didn't help develop good relationships with people. It isolated me more. Therefore I was not really able to help people either. So I wanted to get off the chair, step down and be with the people I wanted to connect with. But I found it very difficult to get down. I had a great fear that if I got down and stopped being Jesus Christ I would not stay in the middle and just be Gary Platz – able to connect with people – but would go straight across the stage, lie down and be powerless, impotent.

I talked to God, who said it was up to me. I could choose not to be Jesus Christ. (This was actually a big part of my 'psychosis'. God gave me free choice. I could stop being Jesus Christ if I wanted. I had free rein to do whatever I thought was right.) I chose someone else to take the part of being me, standing in the middle being just Gary Platz, enjoying connecting with people. But still, I wouldn't come down. Eventually, after much coaxing, I came down and stood in the middle. When I did this, the part of me that was lying down and being powerless ran over and grabbed me and tried to stop me, saying: 'It isn't safe to trust and develop relationships with people. It got you into trouble when you were young. You got sexually abused. I am protecting you.'

After much convincing by interaction with the three roles, I made connections. I enjoyed meeting with and connecting with people, just as *Gary Platz*. I felt safe doing it. Some of the learning from that drama about my 'psychotic experience' was:

* I did not have to become superhuman (Jesus Christ) to be able to have good relationships with people – actually trying to become something extra interfered with relationships.
* Becoming Jesus Christ didn't help me work with people or do the things I wanted to do (I have actually found that I am doing those things now being just me).
* I didn't revert back to being in my worst possible state of powerlessness by relaxing and stopping my striving to be perfect.
* I feel that God accepts me and approves of me. I am still finding a sense of who I am before I develop a stronger relationship with the spiritual.
* People warm to me when I am just Gary Platz.

On the face of it this learning may not seem very much. But when it is put into the context of how entrenched my view of self was, it showed how something extraordinary was needed to make a shift. I was at a point that I could not continue how I was before, in spiritual crisis. I believed in the spiritual but there didn't seem to be anyway that I could trust or feel safe with it. My whole sense of trust in intimacy was abused when I was young. I had to take something extraordinary to gain that trust again. I just could not remain behind those masks anymore and keep living. For me *it took insanity to do it.*

Now I am in a position where I can use the knowledge of my experience to work with others who are finding their way through the awesome lands of madness.

PART FIVE
In the Long Shadow –
In the Light

How poor are they who have not patience!
What wound did ever heal, but by degrees?

Shakespeare

Beginningless time and the present moment are the same. You have only to
understand that time has no real existence.

Huang-Po

I saw Eternity the other night,
Like a great ring of pure and endless light,
All calm, as it was bright;
And round beneath it, Time in hours, days, years,
Driv'n by the spheres
Like a vast shadow mov'd; in which the world
And all her train were hurl'd.

Henry Vaughan

CHAPTER 15

Finding Ourselves by Getting Lost

PHIL BARKER AND POPPY BUCHANAN-BARKER

Who is the 'I' who is 'me'?

> Discovered in her effects, was a photograph of a small boy, on the back of which my mother had written, in pencil, 'Philip aged 4'. I had no recollection of the picture being taken, although it looked like me. The boy was similar to other photographs of 'Philip' with which I was more acquainted. As I turned the picture, back and forth, I wondered if the fact that she had written my name in pencil, and it was therefore amenable to editing, was of any significance. I came to no conclusions.

We use the story of an old snapshot – a very common story indeed – to explore our understanding of 'me', my 'self' and 'I'. Given that the photograph is attributed to someone, this attributed reality raises the issue of who is the 'I' who claims ownership of the 'me' in the photograph? More specifically, anyone can reasonably ask, to what extent can 'I' (present) claim ownership of 'me' (past)? We might go further and ask: to what extent can we claim ownership of anything in a human universe characterized by flux; a universe that is constantly moving, shape shifting, incessantly changing?

The 'I' that was the boy 'Phil' is separate, in space and time, from the 'me' that the man Phil sees depicted in the photograph. Given that this is a found object, the *I* and the *me* we are discussing are not even related by memory, or at least not by any specific memory of the taking of the events surrounding the photograph. It could be said that I (Phil) am not the same *person* that I was when the picture was taken. This begs the questions how the 'me' (of the boy Phil) came to be 'I' (of the man Phil), and into what 'I' (Phil as he is now) am becoming at this moment?

This kind of question has been asked in different ways down at least the past three hundred years and doubtless across many cultures. It was posed in an informative and interesting fashion by Alan Watts in *Beyond Theology*, when he portrayed the *acquisition* of knowledge – if indeed knowledge can be acquired, like goods – as being like a Chinese box. He coyly observed that, 'Whoever *knows* that he knows must be amazed' (Watts, 1973: 3). He added that the possibility of *both* knowing *and* being would involve us in losing ourselves in a maze. 'Knowing that one knows,' Watts said, involves, of necessity, the generation of a confusion of echoes in which, the original sound is lost. 'When "I" know that "I" know, which one', begged Watts, 'is "I": the first that knows, or the second that knows that I know, or the third that knows that I know that I know?' Although already fascinating, this riddle does not even begin to mirror the reflections involved in begging the question, 'who is the "I" who is "me"?'

Watts' echoes of the self suggest something of the poetics of everyday personal experience, which Thomas Szasz has called the *autologue* (Szasz, 1996: ix). 'We' (whoever we are) engage in diverse dialogues with our 'private' selves (whatever they might be). We are interested only in asking these philosophical questions for a practical purpose: what do such questions *mean*, especially within the sociocultural constructions of *mental* health and illness?

Reasoning about madness

These poetics (I-me-myself-mine) provide a useful echo of the corridors of madness, where all manner of disaffected and disoriented individuals wander in search of their identities, if not, actually, in pursuit of their fleeting selfhood. The archetypal lunatic – reduced today to someone with a '*serious and/or enduring mental health problem*' – is classically bereft of reason. How we establish the extent to which people are 'reason deficient', or how they manage to be 'continually' (enduringly) in such a state, is unclear. Yet reason, or the mechanism by which persons express it, remains the central measure of the polarized states of sanity and madness. Reason, at least in the traditional European canon, is the rudder of the functional mind. Without reason we are cast adrift, and soon lose not just our sense of direction, but also our sense of how, if not why, we set sail in the first place.

Today, it is increasingly commonplace to defer all consideration of Watts' dilemma on the grounds that the mind is the location of the 'I' and the mind is located (and constructed by) the brain. Consequently, Watts' dilemma becomes redundant.

The neuroscientific discourse is of critical relevance to our consideration of madness, since people in the grip of madness are entrapped in a consideration of selfhood that many of us avoid. Madness often involves the perennial existential crisis: who am I? And what, on earth, am I doing here? This is not to say that other things are not involved in the construction of this human crisis – signposts, en route to the ultimate concerns the person will express about her or his 'selfhood'. However, the *core* crisis involves the person's presumed relationship with Self, albeit by dint of some troublesome relations with the Other. Given that this relationship is with something that is abstract, invisible, shifting and – in the case of Phil's old photo – embedded in the distant past, we would call this a spiritual relationship.

Vanishing the mind

People were described, carelessly and variously, as 'mentally ill' or '*suffering* from a mental illness', until Thomas Szasz (1961) drew attention to the obvious metaphorical allusion involved. With the increasing politicization of mental health, especially the emergence of the user/consumer advocacy movement, many have taken issue with the implied passivity involved in 'suffering' from mental illness, as well as with the problematic nature of the presumed 'illness' itself, which, like a psychic body-snatcher, somehow takes over the personhood of the individual temporarily or, in the contemporary parlance of the 'enduringly mentally ill', occupies the person indefinitely. Although Szasz's view has frequently been caricatured as a denial of the existence of mental distress, even a casual reading of his considerable output reveals this to be fallacious. Perhaps more than any other modern commentator on the human condition, Szasz has consistently asked what *exactly* was being expressed through the increasingly medicalized language of psychiatry (Szasz, 1993). People described as mentally *sick* are clearly *ill at ease* with themselves and their world of experience. However, the sickness no more reflects the presence of a disease than is evident in a sick *joke*. Similarly, we talk of the built environment suffering from sick building *syndrome*, or the rusting iron rods within concrete producing a 'concrete *cancer*'. It is accepted that these are no more than metaphorical allusions. Yet the 'sickness' that affects the 'mind' is still thought to be a function of some invisible force that (perhaps) rots away the reason of the person from within.

By promulgating Harry Stack Sullivan's conception of mental illness – especially psychosis – as a *problem of living* (Sullivan, 1953), Szasz helped clarify the social, interpersonal and especially moral dimensions of the experience of what once was simply known as madness. We can no more have a blue feeling than we can have a sick mind. Despite the excitement over reports of positron emission computerized tomography (PET scans) 'lighting up the parts of the brain' when people are 'hallucinating', this merely suggests that we have captured a highly focused image of the brain 'at work'. The idea that we might ever capture completely the phenomenon of 'schizophrenia', in form and meaning, is akin to suggesting that we could photograph a dream.

Psychiatrists always were great conjurors, who with great dramatic flourishes, not to mention sleight of hand, would conjure an 'illness' out of thin air. Now they appear to be crafting the 'great mind disappearing trick'. In the physicist John Polkinghorne's 'mind' this betrays considerable conceit:

> We have to be realistic enough, and humble enough, to recognise that much of what is needed for eventual understanding is beyond our present grasp.
>
> Polkinghorne (1996: 73)

Contemporary psychiatric/mental health practitioners continue to reify the notion of mental *illness*, but increasingly, in practice, talk of mental *disorders* (American Psychiatric Association, 1994). This suggests that the psychiatric establishment has quietly capitulated to Szasz's examination of the social and interpersonal context of personhood, which carried implicit questions about our understanding of the nature and meaning of being human in general, and how this was a function of various social, political and especially legal forces. The notion of a mental or psychiatric *disorder* carries the implication that *order* is both naturally occurring and a good thing. By 'good' I mean that it is something to be pursued, with the natural corollary that 'disorder' needs not only to be diminished, but also eliminated.

The implication that people with 'mental illness' are disordered – out of step with social mores – frequently has betrayed the oppressive nature of some social and cultural institutions, which in turn have, traditionally, disenfranchised and pathologized minority groups (e.g. homosexual persons). What society in general cannot countenance (as was the case with homosexuality), or what makes others uncomfortable (e.g. people talking 'as if' they are possessed by aliens or demons), merits classification as a 'disorder' (Kirk and Kutchins, 1997). Apart from the obvious fact that this is no more than a normative position, it implies that there is a 'right and proper' way to *live* with others (socially) and to *be* with ourselves (experientially). Forty years ago Laing noted the irony inherent in Western society classifying unusual, but relatively benign, forms of behaviour as abnormal, when much more malign conduct – towards self or others – was accommodated, if only by convention (Laing, 1967). Today a new generation of psychiatrists are expressing their unease at the blinkered vision of biomedicine (Double, 2002) or how medical training seeks to instil assumptions about 'treatment', which requires patients to adjust themselves to fit 'into an addictive, sexist, racist, self-destructing society' (Schaeff, 1992).

Increasingly, political correctness has challenged the disenfranchising effects of pejorative labelling, substituting its own label of 'persons with mental health problems'. This saccharine-sweet euphemism throws occupational stress and suicidal despair into the same portmanteau. Similarly, this implies that mental health is a birthright, rather than a social construction, and that some people acquire, or otherwise encounter, a problem in maintaining their access to this natural state. This assumption glosses over the rather obvious fact that health and illness are mercurial phenomena. Neither appears to be, at best, anything more than a passing experience. This raises the crucial question that lies at the heart of this address – who am I? When 'I' am disturbed, or disordered, does this also involve a disturbance and disorder of 'me'?

The problem of 'the problem'

Alvarez (1971) traced the origins of the concept of the mental health *problem* to the USA where, in his view, all problems were seen as phenomena in search of a solution. The problems that we experience may not be with this abstract idea of our 'health', but with something more tangible. Maybe the problems we experience involve our *engagement* with life and the necessary processes involved in living. But what, exactly, is the nature of this engagement? Who (or what) is engaging, in what way, with what (or whom)?

Harry Stack Sullivan popularized the contemporary notion that we (and our lives) might be problematic in an intertwined sense when, almost 70 years ago, he began to frame 'mental illness' or 'psychiatric disorder' as a 'problem of living' (Evans, 1996). In Sullivan's view, the problems that people experienced – which others called madness, or mental illnesses, like schizophrenia – were primarily problems experienced as a function of living. More specifically, Sullivan saw people commonly classed as mentally ill – but especially those defined as psychotic – as having problems in their relationships, or dealing with themselves, with others or with the world in general. From this simple observation, he developed a complex, but elegant, theory of interpersonal relations, which proposed not only ways of making sense of how such 'problems of living' might have developed, but also how they might be remedied, or otherwise resolved (Sullivan, 1953).

In his original writings, Sullivan anticipated some of the propositions of postmodern therapists, especially those who emphasized the linguistic power of the narrative, when he drew attention to the way people *construed* (constructed) these problems of living, through the stories they told themselves or others about their lives, and their experiences in living. More recently, Jenner et al. (1993) redrew some of the sociocultural, or even political, boundaries of states that we call schizophrenia; acknowledging that such states may be no more and no less than 'ways of *being or becoming human*'.

By attributing 'problem' status to any experience, we assume that something *needs* to be done or, more importantly, that something *can* be done. In discussing his own attempted suicide, Alvarez poignantly observed that he might have been entrapped by the 'American dream' that all problems have solutions when, in retrospect, he realized that his 'problem' was his life, which was not amenable to such 'fixing'. Alvarez (1971: 282) wrote:

> The despair that had led me to try to kill myself had been pure and unadulterated, like the final, unanswerable despair a child feels, with no before and after. And childishly, I had expected death not merely to end it but also to explain it. Then, when death let me down, I gradually saw that I had been using the wrong language; I had translated the thing into Americanese. Too many movies, too many novels, too many trips to the States had switched my understanding into a hopeful alien tongue. I no longer thought of myself as unhappy; instead, I had 'problems'. Which is an optimistic way putting it, since problems imply solutions, whereas unhappiness is merely a condition of life, which you must live with, like the weather. Once I had accepted that there weren't ever going to be any answers, even in death, I found to my surprise that I didn't much care whether I was happy or unhappy: 'problems' and 'the problem of problems' no longer existed. And that in itself is already the beginning of happiness.

Doing something by doing nothing

Although written over 30 years ago, Alvarez's treatise on suicide anticipated the spiritual inquiry that has gripped the mental health field, in general, over the past decade. Alvarez recognized that human life had always been 'problematic'. Increasingly, however, many people who describe themselves as having 'recovered' from some of the psychiatric/psychological states viewed as 'serious forms of mental illness' (Deegan, 1988) often avoid the use of the popular 'problem-solving' language. Indeed, some emphasize the galvanizing effect of such problems or the necessary nature of such life difficulties, for their human growth and development (Barker et al., 1999). These contemporary views echo Alvarez's epiphany encountered at the cusp of life and death called suicide.

However we view problems of living, we are drawn to consider how we might explore what *needs to be done* (Reynolds, 1983) to live with, resolve or otherwise address the problem. In some cases, what needs to be done may be (literally) nothing. Passive awareness (if indeed this is an *in-action*) can sometimes be the most desirable course of action. This appeared to be the wisdom ultimately revealed to Alvarez. In other cases, some kind of active response to the problem may be developed, but the target of any such action is not so much a moving target as an illusory phenomenon. The problem of living is an idea: it is wholly conceptual. Such problems may be experienced as forms of feeling, emotion or thought; they may be sensed as being embedded in the physical body; or they may be perceived as occupying some space between us and the world of others. In all such instances, however, they are linguistic constructions. When we engage people, or ourselves, in an examination of their relationship to their presumed 'inner selves' or 'person', or their relationship with others, the only material 'thing' with which we can connect is the story: the emergent narrative.

The self-constructing self

The interpersonal processes involved in helping people identify and address their problems of living operate, therefore, at the level of a linguistic exchange. The outcome of this exchange – if such a concrete metaphor is not inappropriate – is the re-authoring, retelling or editing of the problem of living.

This prompts us to ask about the necessary boundaries of the therapeutic encounter – especially in psychiatric settings. Traditionally, the body of information collected together to represent the story of the patient is called the *history*. This implies an appreciation of the potential explanatory power of certain past events (as all past events cannot be accounted for) for the person's current situation. This appreciation – well established as a rationale in biomedicine, but also evident in some psychological theories and models – assumes a causal relationship between past and future (the fantasy imagined in the present). It also assumes that the person might *repeat* her or his history.

Hilda Peplau observed in conversation that 'people make themselves up as they talk' (Peplau, personal communication). This implies the constructive nature of the emergent discourse when two or more people engage in discourse. During this process there will be claims to ownership of *my* thoughts or *my* feelings, echoing the substance of *me/mine*. Such ownership is illusory. Perhaps it is fairer to say that we notice certain thoughts, beliefs and feelings as they (metaphorically) pass, belonging neither to us nor our discussant or informant, but merely (wholly) part of our conjoined reality. We deceive ourselves into thinking that we can pick these up, like objects; incorporating them as our own, a part of *our* territory; storing them in our psyche. This appears to be no more than a linguistic operation, breeding metaphor from metaphor in the further construction of the *self* and by implication the *mind*.

Approaching this issue from a non-Western perspective, Doi (1988: 31) noted:

> Words both express and conceal the mind, and so does the face, but these two acts of expression/concealment are not always concurrent. We could even say that one's facial expressions are more honest than words. On the other hand, words provide a much larger quantity of information, though it must also be said that the more there is expressed the more there is that is concealed.

It should not surprise us that Takeo Doi was Japanese, given that his words, like the point he is making, are at one and the same time enigmatic *and* revelatory. The pronoun 'I' in a Japanese sentence is usually not articulated but understood. To hear the word 'I' in Japan is unusual and not the norm as in the West, where 'I' is not only used extensively but also capitalized. Japanese people may not refer to *themselves* as 'Mr' or 'Mrs' in any context, but no one would address another person without using such a title. The 'self' is valued in Japan but to a much lesser degree, or perhaps in a very different way.

For the Westerner, many aspects of Japanese society may appear illogical or contradictory. One such dynamic is embodied in the notion of *omote*, the outer or public aspect of a person or group, and *ura*, the inner or private aspect. The concept of *omote/ura* is difficult for foreigners, presenting a paradox that resists comprehension. To borrow a weak Western metaphor, *omote/ura* are two sides of the same coin, opposing yet protecting each other.

Doi's appreciation of the relations between inner and outer bears only a superficial resemblance to Western notions of phenomenon and essence. Through Doi's attempt to capture (linguistically) something of the ineffability of the self, we gain a glimpse of its illusory status. Not only may there not be a True Self (in the sense that it has been pursued in the West), but there may not be *any* self, awaiting discovery 'within' the mirror of our reflection or 'beneath' the scratch we make on the surface of our empirical lives. Our selves may be the conjunction of opposites, like *omote/ura*, or even self/no-self (Brandon, 2000).

In everyday life we *conceptualize* the world of experience. This is not *experience* (per se) but, rather, is the second-hand account of that experience. Indeed, when we ask ourselves questions about our experience of the world we cannot (literally) conceive of *it* (experience) without conceptualizing, framing linguistically the 'it' of experience. More critically, in a social context, we employ standardized concepts as part of the carpentry. In principle, it is possible to create a new concept and then to use this to build the frame for our experience. Typically, however, we employ the ready-made frame – using the 'ready-mades' available in the vernacular. However, increasingly we use professional jargon to frame our more awkward experiences, especially those almost-invisible conceptions that appear to lie just beyond our awareness (Rogers, 1995).

Here we are considering some of the experiences that might embody our presence in the world. We appear to be asking, 'How do I know I am here?' As Descartes quizzed himself in a similar vein he wrote:

> 'I noticed that while I was trying to think everything false, it must needs be that I, who was thinking this, was something. And observing that this truth, I am thinking, therefore I exist (Je pense, donc je suis) was so solid and secure that the most extravagant suppositions of the sceptics could not overthrow it, I judged that I did not scruple to accept it as the first principle of [the] philosophy that I was seeking.'

Williams (1972: 347)

Although Descartes has been blamed for the whole mind–body split that has bedevilled human affairs, but especially psychology, in Szasz's view this is mistaken.

> Instead, it would be more accurate to view him as a pioneer neuromythologist, the first to have claimed to have discovered evidence for locating the soul inside the cranium.

Szasz (1996: 107)

Perhaps Descartes' first mistake was to begin his 'search' with the assumption that 'I' existed. But, as Hagen (1995) asked, what did Descartes mean? 'Does he mean his *mind* is thinking? Does he mean his *body* is thinking? *Who* (or perhaps *what*) is doing the thinking here?'

The Ghost in the Machine

Through this assumption Descartes trapped his homuncular self at the end of an infinite regression and, as Hagen noted, we cannot get to it (Hagen, 1995:45). If we change subjects we could just as easily say that:

> *It* is raining therefore *it* is!

Are we assuming that there is some 'thing' that is 'doing' the raining? Some thing that is, in some essential, primary sense, separate from the rain itself?

The challenges of dualism are still with us. It is a warm day and we are relaxing in the garden when a visitor from Mars 'beams in'. We are drinking tea from our best china cups and our new friend, the alien anthropologist, asks, 'What is "it" that we are doing?'. In an attempt to simplify things we say that we are drinking some special water. And so he asks (incorrigibly) what is water? We could answer by simply handing him the cup and saying 'try some'. But today we are working too hard, and we begin to offer an explanation. 'It is hydrogen and oxygen.' Still dissatisfied he asks, 'What is "hydrogen" and "oxygen"?' Vainly, we explain that hydrogen is an element made of atoms, each consisting of a single proton and a single electron. Now he is getting very interested: 'What is a proton ... ?' And so we journey to the limits of our understanding of physics (which is not too far anyway) as we map in finer and finer detail some*thing*, but all the time we are moving further and further away from the original question: 'What is water?' The name, clearly, is not the thing, just as the map, clearly, is not the territory (Korzybski, 1933).

Is this cup of water a metaphor for the self? Perhaps. Let us consider another cup. In his famous elliptical take on the life journey, Lao Tzu wrote:

> What is a vessel? If you take clay and shape it into a vessel, the function of the clay lies in the space which is absent of clay.
>
> Lao Tzu (1995: Chapter 11)

The Western mind, traditionally, perceives a paradox, or contradiction (rightfully), in the space defining the cup and the cup being defined by its absent 'self' (the space). In human terms 'I' *am* what I am not. If we extend our reflection, we may consider the thoughts that *imagined* the cup, the hands that *shaped* the cup, the wheel that set the clay *spinning* through the hands, the hands that *dug* the clay from the ground, the various living things that died and crumbled to form the clay, and so on back through time. Can we separate all this thinking, acting, ingenuity and skill from what we call 'the cup'? Where, metaphorically, do we draw the line that might distinguish the cup from everything that is not the cup? What happens if we apply this anti-logic to our consideration of the 'self'?

Are we giving birth to – constructing or creating – an idea of cup-ness, or cup-hood, which is unreal in the accepted sense? If we ask the same question about the self and its 'self-hood', are we not engaged in as similarly futile pursuit?

Whenever we talk of believing, conjecturing, considering, contemplating, deliberating, presuming, meditating, musing, pondering, reasoning, reflecting, ruminating, supposing, surmising and of course *thinking*, we refer to various conversations with the self – the *autologue* as Tom Szasz called it, or 'talking to yourself' as it was known to our working class parents. But what, or whom – exactly – is talking to what (or whom)? To the Zen Master the answer is to laugh.

In psychiatry, what is *actually* going on remains an issue of key concern, if only to a minority. Szasz noted how the Renaissance idea of the 'malady' had been employed to explain how the minds of self-murderers were 'attacked'. This led to the idea that anyone who (mis)behaved was experiencing a disease of the mind, which today has been translated into a 'chemical imbalance' that causes (putatively) neurotransmitters to malfunction. However, as Szasz continues:

> It makes no more sense to suggest that the brain can be held responsible for homicidal or suicidal acts, than to hold the lung responsible for self-suffocating asthma.
>
> Szasz (1996: 46)

Where does this take us (or leave us) when we consider the 'self' that suffers a collapse of esteem, an injury or a sudden rush of 'consciousness'?

I remember me

When we play with our experience of 'self' we play with memory. In making sense of where we are *now*, we are preparing for the next ontological step – deciding where we move to next. The proposition that memory is located in the brain is absurd. A person with a hearing deficit would not say that memory is located in the ears – far less the brain. Memory for such a person is more likely to be located in the fingers, the medium of communication about everyday, moment-to-moment experience. Memory, like mind, is not an entity located in space (Szasz, 1996). Memory is a narrative that people create from moment to moment, as we engage with our world of experience. We create and often correct or recreate it.

Despite our efforts to get down to the essence of things, including people, it would appear that we only understand the world in terms of its function or our relationships with it, and the people in it. Consciousness, as Hagen (1995) noted, donates the idea of 'thingness' to things. It – *consciousness* – is the source of ideas and things. *It* breaks down Reality into little pieces, splitting the Whole into conceived objects. It does this with the self, conceiving a self that is opposed to everything else, spuriously creating a bogus sense of self-consciousness. What 'it' does not tell us is that, by implication, the self must be everything that it is not, in the spirit of *ura/omote*.

The view of Reality and the construction of the self, which we have examined here all too superficially, is important for the field of mental health, where self-hood and self-consciousness are assumed to be key actors. Much of the current state of play in the field is focused on mechanisms (albeit metaphorical in the Szazsian sense) that might allow or help people to use their 'I' to manage or contain or control 'me'. This is the case especially within the domain of what is called the cognitive behavioural modality of therapy: the assumption that parts of the self can manage, contain or change other parts of the self are powerfully holding the centre ground of practice (viz. self-*management*, self-*control*, self-*instructional training*). These purport to offer an explanation of how change occurs, although in our view this is illusory, and not just because it is philosophically weak. It also appears weak in terms of our physical existence. As we noted at the outset, our difficulty in perceiving the self is partly physical and partly linguistic, although in actuality they cannot be distinguished.

Since we are physical beings, presumably we obey the laws of the physical universe. When taking tea I lift the cup from the table to my lips. It moves from position A to position B. That the cup *can* move is obvious. This is a commonsense assumption. However, as Hagen has asked, how can a commonsense object – like a cup – remain the *same*, remain *itself*, and yet move through time and space? How can something endure, persist, abide, retain its identity *and* yet change? Once the cup has moved – from the table to my lips – it is no longer the same object. Yet we conceive of it as the same object. We conceive of it as exactly the same at both points in time and space.

The spiritual story of 'I' and 'me'

Jung told a story about Pueblo Indians who believed that they were sons of the sun. More importantly, they believed that it was their daily duty to perform a ritual that would help their father to traverse the sky. They recognized the onerous nature of this responsibility, something that they did, effectively, not just for themselves but for the benefit of the whole world. This story brought Jung a realization of his own:

> I then realised on what the 'dignity', the tranquil composure of the Individual Indian, was founded. It springs from his being a son of the sun; his life is cosmologically meaningful, for he helps the father and preserver of all life in his daily rise and descent. If we set against this our own self-justifications, the meaning of our own lives as it is formulated by reason, we cannot help but see our poverty.

Jung (1963: 236–267)

This also reminds us how the dead hand of science has impoverished us. Alfred North Whitehead (1967) took a dim view of the effects of subtle reductionism, which reduced the complete world of joyful, exhilarating, awesome *experience* to a world of 'its'. It became, for Whitehead, 'a dull affair, soundless, scentless, colourless; merely the hurrying of material, endlessly, meaninglessly'.

Although some people find the pragmatic interventions of contemporary medicine and psychotherapy helpful, at least in the short term, many people find that they offer only the crudest understandings of what it is to be human. Even the traditional approach of psychoanalysis, which explored the dynamic 'depths' of the unconscious mind, still clung to a largely biological view of our humanity. The richness of our imagination and the sheer breadth of our emotions – stretching from tragic farce to heavenly bliss – are largely ignored. Certainly, our instinct to fulfil ourselves, in a wide variety of ways, and to achieve a sense of connection with the wider universe of consciousness, is missed in its entirety. We might well argue that, viewed from the holistic perspective, the 'old psychology' that underpins psychiatry and much 'mental health' work is less than human, ignoring our capacity for everyday genius, our inherent complexity and eccentricity, and our sense of *soul-fulness*.

Of course, many of our colleagues in mainstream psychology, and especially psychiatric medicine, have argued with us that 'who we are' is essentially brain-based. However, although consciousness, meaning and imagination (to name but a few of our human dimensions) may be expressed through the brain, this is not quite the same as saying that they either belong to the brain or are wholly a function of the brain. Clearly the characters, dialogue and story line of a television play are expressed through the complex electronics of television. However, only a very young child would want to open up the back of the set in search of the characters and the scenery of their lives.

Should we become more like the Pueblo Indians? Would everyday life grind to a halt if each of us began to feel a sense of connection with the earth and the sun, and introduced this into our everyday stories about who and what we are? Perhaps it would, but it would be no more 'unreal' than saying, simply, that 'I' am a product of my gene pool and various random events that occurred during my life on earth. The practice of psychiatry – but especially the field of 'mental health' – might well be enriched by storytelling that reveals something of the genuine riches of our experience of being alive in what appears to be an organized but random universe.

Finding ourselves – and our place in the world

We have a strong sense of origin, although this does not necessarily translate easily into words. The ground beneath our feet is, literally, the ashes of our ancestors. Perhaps for this reason we have a deep appreciation of the struggle for land reclamation rights, expressed by all peoples who have been the subject of colonization. One simple way that we might help our children to respect the land is to remind them of its 'riches', beaten by the feet and splashed by the blood of those who walked and fell, long before we ever came upon it. In a very important sense, we are *of* the earth and, therefore, are innately connected to it. We do not, however, *own* it. Rather, it owns us. Those who would seek to 'reclaim' the land are seeking, at least spiritually, the freedom of the fullest expression of their connection with the land, which bore them, which nurtured them and which affords them the fundamental link with their deepest human history.

The land can be a physical place where we locate our 'selves', although this is a spiritual relationship, since the 'I' of ourselves and the 'it' of the land become joined in the spirit of all that lies beyond us. Yet many people often feel a great desire to belong to something outwith themselves – an organization or a group. Here they hope to find themselves. John O'Donohue cautions against such false belonging. Membership is not belonging.

> People need to belong to an external system because they are afraid to belong to their own lives. If your soul is awakened then you realise that this is the house of your real belonging. Your longing is safe here. Belonging is related to longing. If you hyphenate belonging, it yields a lovely axiom for spiritual growth: be-your-longing. Where you belong should always be worthy of your dignity. You should belong first in your own interiority. If you belong there and are in rhythm with yourself and connected to that deep, unique source within, then you will never be vulnerable when your outside belonging is qualified, relativised or taken away.
>
> O'Donohue (1997: 182)

In so-called 'mental health' work, rarely is attention paid to the 'interior' – the potential source of strength, and the seedbed of 'personal growth', that lie nestled deep within. Instead, attention is often focused on the management of relationship, of bureaucratic membership – of clubs, therapy groups and other places in which to 'spend time'. When the person is safely attached to such 'surface belonging', the professional may well feel more secure – at least in the knowledge that, for at least some time, the patient/client/user 'belongs' to someone or something else, and is in 'safe hands'. Such social settings may, ultimately, provide the necessary emotional security for the person to feel able to step into their own interior, and to find belonging within her- or himself. Often, however, if driven by the needs of professionals, society or any well-intentioned 'other', such forms of membership may become just another form of dependency.

Keep it messy

It is clear that Phil Barker has moved through a lot of time and space since the picture he found in his mother's effects was taken. Yet, it is assumed that the 'I/me' of Phil Barker remains, endures, albeit changed in several ways. When people say, 'I am not the person I once was', they are 'self-evidently' revealing one of the enigmas of living and being.

These considerations would appear to have some bearing on the practice of offering help to people in the states of serious distress that have been called madness. If we approach such people 'as if' they are fixed objects, we lose the opportunity to explore the Reality of their experience: how they, and all their identifiers, move through time and space *and* remain the same. How they are comfortably 'at home' in their interior, yet inextricably linked to the land of their forbears or numerous past generations, all of whom 'mean' a great deal in their understanding of 'who' and 'what' they are. We can feign cleverness and say this is a 'physical law', but in a simpler sense this is a human fact known to poets down the ages. In his poem 'Among School Children', WB Yeats brought a poetic perspective to the implications of the paradox of self/no-self – *ura/omote*.

> O body swayed to music. O brightening glance.
> How can we know the dancer from the dance?

The powerful relationship between two people implies something that belongs to neither yet, because of their relationship, belongs paradoxically to both; and to both alone. Everyday conversation is dominated by the blending of stories, which (like a fine whisky) frees us to embellish, expand, invent and extend almost to infinity, the story of who we are and what we are becoming. However, we could well ask, as Yeats did, where does the unique, individual, personal 'self' *go* when it blends in with the unique, individual personal 'self' of the other? More importantly, given the creative exchange that takes place, we might ask, does that individual, unique, personal 'self' ever come back?

It occurred to us some time ago that one of the key features of the 'spiritual experience/encounter/journey' was that it often seemed to turn out to be very messy. We wondered if this 'mess' was actually a mirror of the complexity of the universe of experience, in which all these journeys, encounters and experiences *happen*. So far we have come to no real conclusions.

Much of what we have come to understand about ourselves, our lives and our world of experience grows simpler with each passing day. It is true – we are coming to know more and more about less and less. However, that knowledge is riddled with paradoxes. As we have tried to illustrate here, when we try to simplify things, they appear to grow more complicated; however, even that messy finding does not deter us from believing that, at the end of the day, a simple explanation is possible. Perhaps some of the *mess* that we encounter – whether on the traditional spiritual path or the unconventional path of madness – is a function of our trying too hard to solve the problem of life, or of ourselves. The examination and manipulation of the worlds of 'I' and 'me' – far less our many or non-existent spiritual selves – can often become farcical. We can hear Oliver Hardy resigning himself, once again, to the 'fine mess' that his relationship with Stan Laurel has produced. Yet where would Oliver and Hardy *be* without the mess?

We are nagged by the doubt that keeping it messy *is* a necessary part of being and becoming human. *Mess* may be the grease that oils the wheels of our spiritual journey.

References

Alvarez A (1971) The Savage God: a study of suicide. New York: Random House.

American Psychiatric Association (1994) Diagnostic and Statistical Manual of Mental Disorders, 4th edn. Washington, DC: American Psychiatric Association.

Barker P, Campbell P and Davidson B (1999) From the Ashes of Experience: reflections on madness, recovery and growth. London: Whurr.

Brandon D (2000) Tao of Survival: spirituality in social care and counselling. Birmingham: Venture Press.

Deegan P (1988) Recovery: The lived experience of rehabilitation. Psychosocial Rehabilitation Journal XI(4): 11–19.

Doi T (1988) The Anatomy of Self: the individual versus society. Tokyo: Kodansha International.

Double D (2002) Redressing the imbalance. Mental Health Today, September: 25–27.

Evans FB (1996) Harry Stack Sullivan: interpersonal theory and psychotherapy. London: Routledge.

Hagen S (1995) How Can The World Be The Way It Is? An inquiry for the New Millennium into science, philosophy and perception. Wheaton, IL: Quest Books.

Jenner FA, Monteiro ACD, Zagalo-Cardoso JA and Cunha-Oliveira JA (1993) Schizophrenia: a disease or some ways of being human? Sheffield: Sheffield University Press.

Jung CG (1963) Dreams, Memories and Reflections. New York: Random House.

Kirk SA and Kutchins H (1997) Making Us Crazy: the psychiatric bible and the creation of mental disorders. New York: Free Press.

Korzybski A (1933) Science and Sanity. New York: International Non-Aristotleian Society.

Laing RD (1967) The Politics of Experience. New York: Ballantine Books.

Lao Tzu (1995) Lao Tzu's Tao Te Ching (translated by Timothy Freke). London: Piatkus.

North Whitehead A (1967) Science and the Modern World. New York: Free Press.

O'Donohue J (1997) Anam Cara. London: Bantam Press.

Polkinghorne J (1996) Beyond Science: the wider human context. Cambridge: Cambridge University Press.

Reynolds D (1983) Playing Ball on Running Water. London: Sheldon Press.

Rogers RS (1995) The psychologization of narrating hard times. Studia Psychologica 37(3): 180–182.

Schaeff AW (1992) Beyond Therapy: beyond science. San Francisco: Harper.

Sullivan HS (1953) The Interpersonal Theory of Psychiatry. New York: WW Norton and Co.

Szasz TS (1961) The Myth of Mental Illness: foundations of a theory of personal conduct. New York: Hoeber-Harper.

Szasz TS (1993) A Lexicon of Lunacy: metaphoric malady, moral responsibility, and psychiatry. Brunswick, NJ: Transaction.

Szasz TS (1996) The Meaning of Mind: language, morality and neuroscience. Westport, CT: Praeger.

Watts A (1973) Beyond Theology: the art of Godmanship. New York: Vintage Books.

Williams B (1972) Descartes. In Edwards P (ed.) Encyclopaedia of Philosophy, vol. 2. New York: Macmillan.

Postscript

Long after we finished writing Chapter 15, we read a book given to us by an old friend in New Zealand, written by his brother and niece. Robert and Joanna Consedine's book – *Healing Our History: the challenge of the Treaty of Waitangi* – is a detailed critique of colonization; of how the indigenous people of what became known as New Zealand were exploited, disenfranchised, socially remodelled and in some tragic sense also 'ethnically cleansed' by imperialism. The Treaty of Waitangi represents a structured attempt, in Robert and Joanna's terms, to 'heal history'. It is a project focused, unashamedly, on *understanding*, which often requires us to face very different versions of the 'reality' that we have known or chosen, and which requires us to be responsible, not just for ourselves in the here and now, but perhaps also for those who have gone before us, and in whose name and footsteps we walk.

At the end of their book, Robert wrote:

> I remember with gratitude the Sisters who taught me as a child to see my life in the light of eternity. They enabled me to view my journey as a continuum in relationship to my ancestors. The philosophy I absorbed has profoundly influenced me to make constructive choices in a world where hunger, war, racism, poverty, despair and hopelessness exist. Yet, for me, the paradox of hope remains. I have always managed to maintain faith in my own humanity and a belief in the divine spark in every human being. This hope is constantly nurtured in my relationship with my family, community and a network of people throughout New Zealand and other parts of the world. Maintaining faith when you don't know the reality of suffering can be relatively straightforward. Maintaining faith when you do is the challenge.

> Consedine and Consedine (2001: 230)

Robert and Joanna's book reminds us of the colonization of people with mental illness, many of whom have been exploited, brainwashed, abused and humanly diminished by systems – like imperialism – that claimed to have their 'best interests' at heart. Mental health workers have no 'Treaty of Waitangi' to serve as a guideline, prompt or moral benchmark. Reading their book might help us think of more creative ways to be of help to those dispossessed by mental illness and by the psychiatric system. Reading their book might help us find a way of making an apology to all those who have been colonized by the psychiatric system. Although this might seem to be out of keeping with the overall tone of this book, we believe that making such an apology – in a variety of ways, perhaps as a future 'way of life' in mental health work – would be wholly in keeping with the *spirit* of this book.

Robert's words, in particular, provide a fitting springboard for this post-script. We, too, remember our teachers – extending from our childhood schools, through our families, right up to the present day, but who also include the people we have worked with, who, at least nominally, have been 'in our care'. The old adage, 'when the pupil is ready the master appears', seems so true. We have not always been open to instruction, but we hope that we are ready now. *Now* seems like the best place to begin. *Now* is the beginning and end point of our instruction.

We, too, have been privileged to witness plenty of suffering. We say *privileged*, for so many of the people who have been in great physical or emotional pain looked upon our mere presence as some kind of a blessing, however short-lived. Indeed, our experience of suffering, whether personal or vicarious, has increased our sense of wonder at this simple, often overlooked, fact of life. Often, against all the odds, people do continue to be and become. Our question has long been: 'How do people manage to do that?'

In a world where so many people rush to offer quick fixes, we remain in awe of the legions of people who, somehow or other, have learned how to tap into their sacred interiors and have found the power to live with, or even perhaps to transcend, the distress of their lives. Such people have taught us much about the potential for healing that lies in our relations: with ourselves, as well as with one another; and ultimately with everything of which we are a part.

The Spirit certainly does appear to be among us – even when not obviously within us.

Reference

Consedine R and Consedine J (2001) Healing Our History: the challenge of the Treaty of Waitangi. Auckland: Penguin.

Index